INTRODUCTION

This is the second major update of *The A to Z of the Heart*. Additional organs and their Blood supplies including venous and lymphatic drainage have been added. In conjunction with *The A to Z of Major Organs* and *The A to Z of Reproductive and Sexual organs* this book adds a valuable contribution to the understanding of the function of the cardiovascular system and its relationship to the heart function & structure.

The back cover has also been modified. As with all the new editions of *the A to Zs* it now includes an additional **fold over** which serves as a means of identifying the book on the shelf, a fold in / bookmark and a reminder of all the current A to Zs; icons of the their front covers are placed on the inside flap. Hence the spiral binding is preserved, but the book can easily be identified if this **fold over** is placed outward in the bookshelf.

As usual the material may be viewed along with the other A to Zs on the following sites
http://www.aspenpharma.com.au/atlas/student.htm
www.amandasatoz.com

ACKNOWLEDGEMENT

I would like to thank Aspenpharmacare Australia, in particular Greg Lan and Rob Koster, for their continuing support. Richard Clement has been very helpful in providing IT advice and assistance. Thank you to everyone who provided valuable feedback.

DEDICATION

To those things and people who make my heart beat; to my A to Z and all those letters in between.

HOW TO USE THIS BOOK

The structure of *the A to Zs* grows and develops with each new publication. The principle of listing structures in an alphabetical manner has been maintained, in all sections, after first dividing the material into a number of main topics and introducing overviews of the main structures discussed and their clinical applications. The topics in this case are: the Components of the Circulatory System; the Structure of the Heart; the Blood Supply of the organs and tissues in the body; the Major Blood Vessels, their branches and relations; separate circulations, within the cardiovascular system and finally clinical aspects of the cardiovascular system.

Pages of each section are colour coded, and this is reflected in the Table of Contents, which has colour bars separating each section reflecting that section's page colour.

Thank you
A. L. Neill
medicalamanda@gmail.com
BSc MSc MBBS PhD FACBS
ISBN 978-1-921930-16-4

T0319295

Table of contents

THE BLOOD SUPPLY OF...

TABLE OF CONTENTS

MAJOR BLOOD VESSELS SIGNIFICANT BRANCHES & RELATIONS

CIRCULATIONS

CLINICAL ASSESSMENT OF THE HEART & CVS

Abbreviations

a	= artery
A	= atrium, (pl atria) / actions /movements of a joint
ACF	= anterior cranial fossa
AF	= atrial fibrillation
adj.	= adjective
aka	= also known as
alt.	= alternative
AM	= arachnoid mater
ANS	= autonomic nervous system
ant	= anterior
art.	= artery
AS	= Alternative Spelling, generally referring to the diff. b/n British & American spelling
ASD	= atrial septal defect
assoc.	= associated with
AV	= atrioventricular
B	= blood
BBB	= blood brain barrier
bc	= because
BF	= blood flow
BM	= basement membrane
BP	= brachial plexus/blood pressure
bpm	= beats per minute
br	= branch (of a vessel)
BS	= blood supply / blood stream
b/n	= between
cap.	= capillary
c.f.	= compared to
CM	= cardiac muscle
cm	= cell membrane
CMC	= cardiac muscle cells
CNS	= central nervous system
CO	= cardiac output
collat.	= collateral
CP	= cervical plexus
Cr	= cranial
CSF	= Cerebrospinal fluid
CT	= connective tissue
CVA	= cerebrovascular accident = stroke
dist.	= distal
DM	= dura mater
e.g.	= example
EC	= extracellular (outside the cell)
ECG	= electrocardiogram
Gk.	= Greek
H	= hormone(s)
HB	= heart beat
HF	= heart failure
HP	= high pressure
HR	= heart rate

HS	= heart sounds
IC	= intracellular / intercostal
ICS	= intercostal space
IVC	= inferior vena cava
jt(s)	= joints = articulations
L	= left
LA	= Left Atrium
lat.	= lateral
LL	= lower limb
lig	= ligament
LP	= low pressure
Lt.	= Latin
MCL	= mid clavicular line
med.	= medial
MI	= myocardial infarction
N	= nerve
NS	= nervous system/nerve supply
NT	= nervous tissue
nv	= neurovascular bundle
P	= pressure
PAD	= peripheral artery disease
PaNS	= parasympathetic nervous system
pl.	= plural
PM	= pia mater
PN	= peripheral nerve
post.	= posterior
proc.	= process
prox.	= proximal
R	= Right
RA	= Right atrium
RA	= regarding/in reference to
S	= sacral/sound
S1	= first heart sound
S2	= second heart sound
SA	= sinoatrial
sing.	= singular
SC	= spinal cord
SN	= spinal nerve
SR	= sarcoplasmic reticulum
subcut.	= subcutaneous
supf	= superficial
SS	= signs and symptoms
SVC	= superior vena cava
SyNS	= sympathetic nervous system
T	= thoracic
UL	= upper limb, arm
V	= vertebra / ventricle
VC	= vertebral column
WM	= white matter
w/n	= within
w/o	= without
wrt	= with respect to
&	= and

Common Terms used in Cardiology / Vascular anatomy

Ablation - surgical or catheter scarring of cardiac tissue.

Accessory Pathway - alternative connecting pathway b/n the A & the V - besides the bundle of His resulting syndrome is – Wolf-Parkinson-White syndrome

Actin - one of the 2 contractile fibres of the cardiac & skeletal muscle - the "thin" filament (see also Myosin)

Action Potential - electrical activities of a cell from depolarization to repolarization (5 phases 0-5) involving Calcium, Potassium and Sodium ions

Adrenergic mimicking receptors of the sympathetic NS - adrenaline opposite of cholinergic

Afterload - P needed by the V to eject blood - in the R this is small (the pressure around 30mmHg) - the diastolic pressure of the pulmonary trunk - in the L it is the diastolic P of the aorta + peripheral resistance

Amplitude - the height/depth of the waves in an ECG in mm

Anastomosis - the surgical connection of separate or severed tubular hollow organs to form a continuous channel. - a series of interconnecting blood channels allowing for several directions of BF so that B can reach tissue despite blockages

Aneurysm - a localized dilatation of an artery or heart chamber caused by disease or weakening of the muscle in the wall - tunica media.

Angina / Angina Pectoris - chest pain or discomfort due to lack of oxygen - anoxia or ischemia in the muscle tissue (myocardium) generally bc of coronary artery disease. Angina is a symptom of a condition called myocardial ischemia. May also manifest as : aching, burning, discomfort, heaviness, numbness, pressure, tightness, &/or tingling in the chest, back, neck, throat, jaw or arms.

Angiography - an X-ray that uses dye injected into arteries so that coronary artery anatomy can be studied wrt disease diagnosis. Coronary angiography is done during a cardiac catheterization. see also angiograms

Angioplasty - an insertion of a balloon at the end of a catheter, blown up to compress the clogged area of the artery against the arterial wall and so dilate the lumen which is then removed.

Anticoagulants - also known as: "Blood thinners"; medications that slow blood clotting time. Anyone on anticoagulants needs regular blood tests to determine clotting time eg. Prothrombin time = PT = Protime.

Aorta - the largest artery in the body and the primary BV leading from the heart to the body.

Aortic Valve - the valve that regulates BF from the heart to the aorta.

Apex - (of the Heart) the inferior aspect or bottom of the heart 5th ICS, L MCL, where the HB is the strongest

Arrhythmia - lack of rhythm or HB, abnormal heartbeat (= Dysrthymia), caused by a disruption of the normal functioning of the heart's electrical conduction system. Normally, contraction is coordinated. Arrhythmias/Dysrhythmias result in ineffective and uncoordinated contractions of the CM causing an irregular pulse, CO, CAD, rheumatic heart disease, BP, acute MI, hyperthyroidism and some medications are associated with the development of arrhythmias. Listed below are the types of arrhythmias

• Fibrillation: can be atrial or ventricular. Ineffective beats. see also fibrillation

• Tachycardia: fast heart beat, usually > 110 bpm.

• Bradycardia: slow heart beat, usually < 50 bpm

Arteriole - small artey

Arteriosclerosis - Commonly called "hardening of the arteries", this includes a variety of conditions that cause artery walls to thicken and lose elasticity. It can occur because of fatty deposits in the inner lining of arteries (atherosclerosis), calcification of the wall of the arteries, or thickening of the muscular wall of the arteries from chronically elevated BP. It also is associated with aging diabetes, hyperlipidaemia & hypertension etc. see also Atherosclerosis

Artery - a BV that carries blood away from the heart.

Asystole - absence of a HB - flat line ECG

Atherectomy also known as: Rotorooter. A procedure that uses a catheter and special cutting or grinding tools to remove plaque from artery walls

Atherosclerosis - a form of arteriosclerosis that is caused by a buildup of plaque &/or fatty deposits in the inner lining of an artery.

Atrial Fibrillation (AF) - a disorder of HR and rhythm in which the heart's 2 small, upper chambers (A) quiver rapidly like a bowl of gelatin and empty blood into the heart's lower chambers (V) in a disorganized manner. This may result in blood pooling and clotting in the A. Causes of AF include dysfunction of the SA node, coronary artery disease, rheumatic heart disease, hypertension and hyperthyroidism.

Atrial Septal Defect (ASD) - an abnormal hole in the wall b/n the R & L atria.

Atrium (pl Atria) - Lt antrum = waiting room – top chambers R & L of the heart - 1/3 of the volume of the V or lower chamber.

AV node - see junction

AV junction - see junction

Base - "of the Heart" top of the heart located in the 4ᵗʰ ICS

"Beta stimulation" - responses come from adrenergic = sympathetic stimulation, 1 the HR, contraction force, 2 the bronchial dilatation

Blood Pressure (BP) - the force or pressure exerted by the heart against the walls of the arteries. When the arterioles (smaller arteries) constrict (narrow), the blood must flow through a smaller "pipe" and the pressure rises. High BP adds to the workload of the heart and arteries.

Optimal BP is < 120/80 mm Hg. High BP = hypertension, >140/90 mm Hg - 120-139/80-89 mm Hg are considered pre-hypertension. Hypertension increases the risk of: angina, athersclerosis, CVA, HF, kidney failure, MI & PAD.

COMMON TERMS

Bradycardia - an abnormally slow HB, usually < 60 bpm opposite of Tachycardia

Bundle of His - a pacemaker (40-60bpm) and part of the cardiac conducting system it transmits the electrical stimulation/depolarization through the AV septum to the R & L Purkinje fibres

Bundle branches - part of the cardiac conducting system = bundle of His + Purkinje bundles R+ L

Bundle-branch Block - an interruption of the cardiac conducting system - Purkinje fibres are insulated to conduct the signal rapidly through the Vs – if either side is blocked the other must travel further and hence depolarization is slower - elongating the QRS complex

Burst - a run of 3 or more ectopic HBs

Calcium Ion Channel - part of the SR enlarged in the heart where Ca2 can efflux &/or influx rapidly to allow for contraction of the CMCs

Capillaries - the smallest vessels b/n arteries & veins. Site of gas and nutrient exchange b/n B and T.

Capture - effective depolarization of the A or Vs by a pacemaker

Cardiac Arrest - the sudden stopping of HBs & respiration – clinical death.

Cardiac Cath or Cardiac Catheterization a catheter is inserted into a BV in the arm or groin (after local anaesthesia) and threaded up to the heart, a dye is injected and X-rays are taken of the heart arteries, to investigate blockages or narrowing of the BVs

Cardiac Output (CO) - the volume of B pumped from the V in 1 min. (generally referring to the LV)

Cardiac Tamponade - excess fluid b/n the parietal and visceral layers of the pericardium - this restricts cardiac contraction SS – jugular distention + diminished difference b/n systolic and diastiolic BPs

Cardioversion - the restoration of normal HB by electrical counter shock or by use of medication.

Cardiomyopathy - a disease or disorder of the CM causing it to lose its pumping strength.

Carotid Artery - major artery of the H&N - from the aorta

Catecholamines - Hs and substances of the symNS = adrenalin + noradrenalin AKA epinephrine + norepinephrine + dopamine

Catheter a thin, flexible tube

Cholesterol - a soft, waxy substance found among the lipids or fats in the BS and in all the body's cells. It forms cm and some Hs. Cholesterol and other fats are transported to in the BS by lipoproteins, and can move in and out of cells bc of their fatty nature. There are several kinds of cholesterols, but the most important are low-density lipoprotein (LDL) considered "bad" cholesterol bc they carry triglycerides, high-density lipoprotein (HDL) considered "good".

Cholinergic - refers to substances containing quaternary ammonium salts

Cholinergic - Hs and substances of the PaNS = acetylcholine antagonists to the sympathetic NS substances   see also catecholamines

Chordae Tendineae - tendons connecting the AV valves with the papillary muscles

Chronotropic - concerning HR

Chrono - time

Complete heart block - A & Vs fire independently

Complex - a collection of waveforms QRS complex or ECG complex

Computed Tomography (CT or CAT scan) - a method of examining body organs by scanning them with X-rays and using a computer to construct a series of cross-sectional scans along a single axis.

Conduction - the process of transporting the depolarization stimulus (electrical stimulus) throughout the heart A ⇨ Vs in a specific pathway or along a N.

Conductivity - the ability to conduct an impulse to another region or another cell

Congenital - existing at birth.

Congestive cardia failure (CCF) - Blood volume coming in is more than that able to be pumped out - leading to fluid backup - backup from the LV results in fluid overload in the lungs - in the RV results in venous fluid retention - swelling of dependent parts such as ankles and sacrum.

Coronary Artery Bypass Graft also known as: CABG, "Cabbage". Surgery done to bypass the blocked coronary artery. Uses a vein from the leg or chest to carry the blood as "a bridge" around the blocked coronary artery.

Coronary Arteries - Two arteries arising from the aorta that arch down over the top of the heart & branch out in additional arteries that provide B to the heart muscle

Coronary Artery Disease (CAD) - Conditions that cause narrowing of the coronary arteries, reducing BF to the CM. Blockage or narrowing may be due to clots, lipids &/or plaques. Severe cases can result in heart attack.

Coronary Artery Bypass Grafting (CABG) - heart surgery in which a section of a BV is grafted to the coronary artery to bypass the blocked section of the coronary artery and improve the BF to the heart.

Defibrillation - the process of depolarizing the whole heart and creating an asystole in order to re-establish a sinus rhythm

Defibrillator - an electronic device used to establish a normal HB.

Depolarization - rapid influx of positive ions across the cell membrane to allow contraction

Dextrocardia - the heart is in the R thorax and chambers are reversed - rare

Diastole - phase of relaxation in the cardiac cycle first A and then Vs lasts up to 2X as long as the systole, allows for the chambers to fill

Dyskinetic - a sub-optimal contracting myocardium due to ischaemia

Dysrhythmia - arrhythmia abnormal rhythm

Echocardiogram - a study using high-frequency sound waves to picture or visualize the heart chambers, the thickness of the muscle wall, the heart valves and major BVs located near the heart. This is a non-invasive procedure.

Echocardiography - the use of ultrasound in the diagnosis of cardiovascular lesions and in recording the size, motion, and composition of various cardiac structures.

Ectopic - wrt the heart a depolarizing wave originating outside the SA node

Ejection Fraction - the measurement of the B pumped out of the Vs compared to the total amount of B in the V (Normal is 60%).

Electrocardiogram (ECC or EKG) - a test that records the electrical activity of the heart, shows abnormal rhythms and detects heart muscle damage (heart attacks), graph of the electrical conduction system of the heart

Electrolytes - elements or chemicals, generally anions or cations, needed to enable the body and heart to work properly. The most frequently tested are: Sodium, Potassium, Calcium & Chloride; levels outside the normal range cause cardiac (heart) and other problems.

Electrophysiological Study (EPS) - a cardiac catheterization to study electrical current in patients who have arrhythmias.

Endocarditis - inflammation of the endocardium generally to infection that may affect heart valves and the aorta.

Endocardium - smooth innermost layer of the heart, covers all chambres and the valves - continuous with the endothelium lining the BV lumen

Endotracheal Tube (ETT) - a tube inserted into the trachea (wind pipe) to provide a passageway for air.

Enzymes AKA cardiac enzymes - term used wrt when there is suspected cardiac muscle damage and cell death - certain enzymes are released from these cells and their levels rise acutely.

Epicardium - the membrane that covers the outside of the heart –fused with the visceral pericardium often used interchangeably with this term, supports the cardiac vessels before they penetrate the myocardium

Excitability - a cells ability to respond to an impulse by depolarizing or by spontaneous depolarization

Extrasystole - premature depolarizating complex or HB

Fibrillation - rapid irregular contractions of the heart muscle.
> *Atrial fibrillation* 350-600 bpm but only a max of 240 bpm can pass through to the ventricles (no P waves - narrow QRS complex)

Flutter - ineffective contractions of the heart muscles.

Heart Attack AKA **myocardial infarction** is the sudden interruption or insufficiency of the supply of blood to the heart, typically resulting from occlusion or obstruction of a coronary artery and often characterized by severe chest pain.

Heart Block - impaired conduction of the impulse that regulates the HB - may cause sudden attacks of unconsciousness.

Heart-lung Machine - a machine that pumps and oxygenates blood during open-heart surgery.

Heart rate - number of QRS complexes on an ECG – note this may not be the same as the pulse rate

Heart Valve Prolapse - a condition of the heart valve in which it is partially open when it should be closed.

His-Purkinje system - the electrical network of fibres which includes the Bundle of His, bundle branches and Purkinje fibres

Hyperkalaemia - increased potassium levels in the B

Hypertension - high BP = diastolic > 90 mmHg and systolic >140 mmHg

Hypokalaemia - decreased potassium levels in the B

Hypotension - low BP = diastolic < 70mg systolic <90 mmHg

Hypoxia - a sub therapeutic B oxygen level resulting in reduced energy production and level of lactic and pyuvic acid (anaerobic metabolism)

Incompetence - re valves indicates a valve which allows regurgitation – backflow of blood

Infarction - cell death due to anoxia

Intravascular Echocardiography - echocardiography used in cardiac catheterization.

Invasive procedure - a procedure, test or surgery that involves going through the skin or muscle or into a vein or artery, such as a Cardiac Catheterization

Ischemia - reduced oxygen supply - in the heart generally refers to reduced BS due to plaque blockage in the coronary arteries.

Ischemic Heart Disease - a disease characterized by reduced BS to the heart.

Junction - as in AV junction b/n the A & the Vs - allows the impulse to go from the A to the Vs, and slows it via the AV node (a supraventricular structure) and the bundles of His. If the sinus does not generate an impulse the AV junction will fire at 40-60 bpm

Left Ventricular Assist Device (LVAD) - a mechanical pumping device that is surgically implanted; it helps maintain the pumping action of the heart and often used in patients who are waiting for a heart transplant.

Lymphatic - a vessel which carries fluid to the heart

MAZE - known as the micro-MAZE, this innovative videoscopic operation offers a surgical remedy for AF w/o opening the chest or stopping the heart. With the micro-MAZE operation, access to the heart is achieved through 3 one - centimeter (keyhole) incisions on each side of the patient's chest.

Mechanical Valves - artificial valves made from metal, plastic, and/or pyrolytic carbon.

Mediastinum - the region in the thorax b/n the lungs, ant. boundary - the sternum post. the VC, includes the heart, roots of the great vessels, oesophagus and trachea.

Microvasculature - the network of small BVs arterioles capillaries venules in a tissue

Minimally Invasive Heart Surgery - a variety of approaches using smaller incisions to reduce the trauma of surgery and potentially speed recovery.

Mitral Valve - the valve that controls the BF b/n the LA & LV in the heart.

Mitral Valve Prolapse - a bulge in the valve b/n the LA & LV of the heart that causes backward flow of the blood into the atrium.

Murmur - a specific sound emanating from the chest in addition to the normal HS.

Myocardial Infarct - also called "heart attack"; the sudden interruption or insufficiency of the supply of B to the heart, typically resulting from occlusion or obstruction of a coronary artery and often characterized by severe chest pain

Myocardial infarction AKA **Heart attack** death of myocardial tissue due to anoxia.

Myocardial Ischemia - insufficient BF to part of the heart.

Myocardium - the muscle of the heart = heart muscle - middle layer responsible for contraction

Myocyte - muscle cell, may be smooth or striated then cardiac or skeletal

Myosin - the "thick" filament of the 2 filaments which bind together in heart muscle contraction (see also Actin)

Nodal - refering to junctional functions

Non-invasive procedure - a procedure that can be done outside of the body, such as an X-ray or ECG. (see also invasive procedure)

NTG-Nitro-Nitroglycerine - a medication that expands or relaxes arteries to enable B to flow more easily. It can be taken by mouth, spray, skin patch, or intravenously

P - wave - wave formed by atrial depolarization

P - R interval - time b/n P wave beginning and the beginning of the QRS complex

Pacemaker - surgically implanted electronic devices used to stimulate or regulate contractions of the heart muscle.

Palpitation - irregular HB that can be felt by a person.

Pericardium - 2X layered sac surrounding the heart filled with 30-50 mls of surfactant

Peripheral Resistance - the obstruction to BF in the body's tissues

Plaque - a build up in the lining of a damaged artery. It can be caused by high B cholesterol, smoking, ↑BP

Prolapse - collapse

Pulmonary Valve - the heart valve located b/n the RV and the pulmonary artery that controls BF to the lungs.

Pulmonary Vein - the vessel that carries newly oxygenated blood to the heart from the lungs.

Pulse - the beat of the heart felt in an artery.

QRS interval - electrical representation of ventricular depolarization

Refractory period - period when the contractile CMCs are not fully repolarized

- absolute refractory period when it is impossible to restimulate the cells due to depolarization no matter how large the stimulating impulse

Regurgitation - is BF in the opposite direction from normal.

Rheumatic Heart Disease - a condition resulting from certain strep infections that occasionally cause disease in the joints & heart valves.

Rhythm - cardiac beating rhythm normally started from the SA node – AKA sinus rhythm (80-120 bpm) - Junctional rhythm when the contraction is started by the AV node generally 60-100 bpm (P waves absent – QRS shortened PR interval inverted see also ECG)

Risk factors - habits or characteristics which can increase the likelihood of developing heart disease.

Non-modifiable risk factors (risk factors that cannot be changed):
- Family history of coronary disease or stroke
- Age
- Sex

Modifiable risk factors (risk factors that can be changed):
- Smoking
- High Blood Pressure (hypertension)
- Diet high in animal fats
- Sedentary lifestyle (couch potato)
- Diabetes
- Stress
- Type "A" personality
- Obesity
- Excessive use of alcohol

Run = burst

Saphenous Vein - a vein on the inside of the leg running from the ankle to the groin that can be used to create bypasses from the aorta to the coronary arteries.

Septal Defect - a congenital abnormality in the septum b/n the L & R Vs.

Septum - the wall that divides the heart chambers.

Semilunar valves - referring to the shape of valves like half moons cups which capture any B wanting to flow backwards found in the atrial valves, veins and lymphatics, CT structure covered with endothelial cells

Sick sinus syndrome - altered sinus rhythm due to fibrous tissue growth and interference around the SA node

Sinoatrial node - SA node area of modified CMCs in upper RA serves as the predominant pacemaker of the heart

Sinus Rhythm - the normal rhythm of the heart (60 to 100 beats per minute).

Stable angina (or chronic stable angina) - refers to "predictable" chest discomfort such as that associated with physical activity or mental or emotional stress. Rest and/or nitroglycerin usually relieve stable angina. vs Unstable angina - Refers to unexpected chest pain and usually occurs at rest. It is typically more severe and prolonged and is due to a BF to the heart caused by the narrowing of the coronary arteries. Unstable angina or acute coronary syndrome should be treated as an emergency

Stenosis - the valve opening has not formed correctly or has become narrowed and inflexible (or stenotic) reducing the ability of the heart to pump blood out efficiently.

Stent - devices that are placed in the artery to keep the inner wall of the artery open. Small metal coil or mesh tube, permanently left in the artery

Sternotomy - a type of incision in the center of the chest that separates the sternum (chestbone) to allow access to the heart.

Synctium - multiple nuclear bag of cytoplasm

Tachycardia - accelerated HR generally >100 bpm opposite Bradycardia

Telemetry Unit - a small transmitter that is used to send information about the heart via radio transmission to healthcare professionals for evaluation.

Transesophageal Echocardiography (TEE) - a diagnostic test in which a probe is passed through the oesophagus, measuring the sound waves that bounce off the heart.

Transmural - wrt heart across the full thickness of the muscular wall

Tricuspid Valve - the heart valve that controls the BF from the RA into the RV.

Troponin - protein of the CMC involved in contraction - if present in the B indicates muscle death

T-wave - representation of ventricular repolarization

U-wave - indicates repolarization of purkinje fibres or hypokalaemia or digoxin or quinidine medication

Vagal maneuver - stimulation of the vagal N to decrease HR and BP may cause fainting

Valve - there are 4 heart valves: mitral, aortic, pulmonary and tricuspid, that act as one-way "doors" between the chambers of the heart.

Vein - a BV which carries B to the heart

Ventricular fibrillation - chaotic disorganized HB from one or more centres in the V - stops or diminishes CO and if uncorrected results in death needs cardioversion to correct

Ventricular Septal Defect - a common congenital heart defect; an abnormal opening in the septum dividing the Vs allows blood to pass directly from the L to the R V; large openings may cause CCF.

Ventricles - lower heart 2 chambres

Notes

Guide to Anatomical Planes and Relations

This is the anatomical position.

A = Anterior Aspect from the front Posterior Aspect from the back used interchangeably with ventral and dorsal respectively

B = Lateral Aspect from either side

C = Transverse / Horizontal plane

D = Midsagittal plane = Median plane; trunk moving away from this plane = lateral flexion or lateral movement moving into this plane medial movement; limbs moving away from this direction = abduction; limbs moving closer to this plane = adduction

E = Coronal plane

F = Median

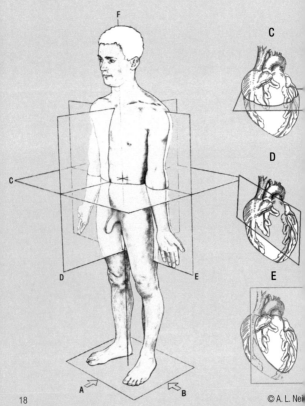

© A. L. Neill

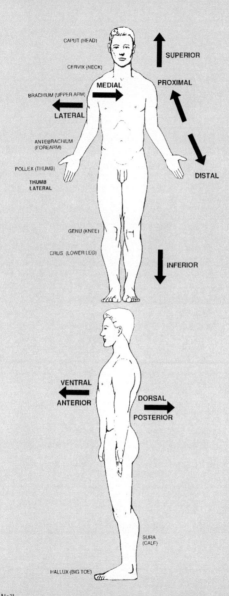

Anatomical Movements

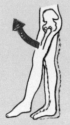

Hip flexion

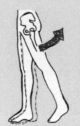

Hip extension

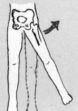

Hip abduction

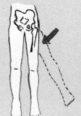

Hip adduction

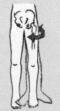

Hip lateral and
medial rotation

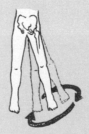

Hip circumduction

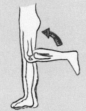

Knee flexion

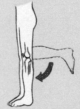

Knee extension

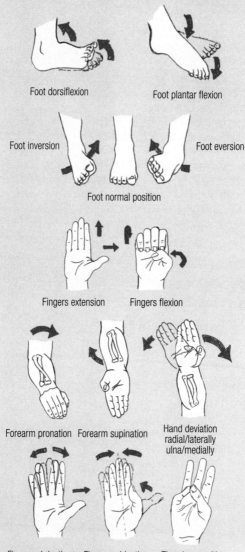

Foot dorsiflexion

Foot plantar flexion

Foot inversion

Foot eversion

Foot normal position

Fingers extension

Fingers flexion

Forearm pronation

Forearm supination

Hand deviation
radial/laterally
ulna/medially

Fingers abduction

Fingers adduction

Thumb opposition

Arteries

Microscopic MP
Large & medium arteries have a similar structure.
They carry B away from the heart.

They maintain an adequate & constant P so B flows rapidly from the heart to tissues, with min. disruption. Hence they have small very smooth lumens (7) lined by tightly connected shiny endothelial cells (1) lying on a BM (2) = THE TUNICA INTIMA. Smooth muscle (4) gives strength to maintain a reasonable R which is further controlled b/n 2 layers of highly elastic tissue (3, 5) minimizing the P differences b/n systole & diastole = THE TUNICA MEDIA. Surrounding CT carries the BVs of the BVs, the vasa vasorum so that the tissues of the BV itself are well nourished. N endings partic. of the ANS are located here so that tone of the BV can be altered- the TUNICA EXTERNA or ADVENTITIA.

1 endothelium
2 basement membrane
3 internal elastic lamina
4 smooth muscle
5 external elastic lamina
6 CT containing fatty tissue / small BVs / Ns
7 lumen

THE TUNICA INTIMA = 1+ 2

THE TUNICA MEDIA = 3 + 4 +5

TUNICA EXTERNA or ADVENTITIA = 6

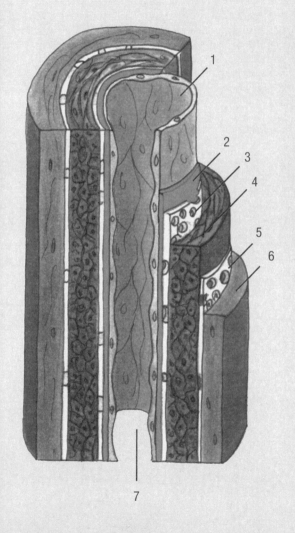

1

2

3

4

5

6

7

Capillaries

Microscopic MP

Capillaries are thin walled BVs designed to allow maximum contact b/n tissue and the oxygen carriers or RBCs. The dimensions are that in most cases the RBCs abut the capillary wall and gases diffuse across according to the concentration gradient. Most capillary beds dilate and fill in anoxic conditions*. Other cells present such as monocytes may palisade along the BV wall or move into the extravascular space, when stimulated.

1 fibrocyte

2 endothelial cell nucleus

3 RBC

4 plasma in capillary

5 surrounding extravascular fluid

6 monocyte in capillary

7 BM

*note pulmonary capillary beds shut down in anoxic conditions

© A. L. Neill

Capillaries

Microscopic MP

Capillary types "normal" *(A)*
Fenestrated *(B)*
Sinusoids *(C)*

Most capillaries have an endothelial cell lining sitting on a protein and fibrous network the BM. The endothelium changes with the function of the tissue. *(A)*

Highly metabolic tissues require large amounts of proteins &/or other substances to be transported via capillaries eg. endocrine glands and intestinal BVs - the endothelium is modified to facilitate this process - widows or fenestrations develop - where the cytoplasm is absent and the cm is the only barrier b/n the lumen and the bm. *(B)*

In the liver and bone marrow, new B cells are made and launched into the BS. To allow cellular transport the bm and endothelium have "holes" - the capillaries are called sinusoids. *(C)*

1 BM
2 endothelial cell nucleus
3 cytoplasm of the endothelium
4 vacuole for transport of substances
5 RBC
6 cell to cell connection in endothelium
7 fenstration
8 gap in endothelium + bm

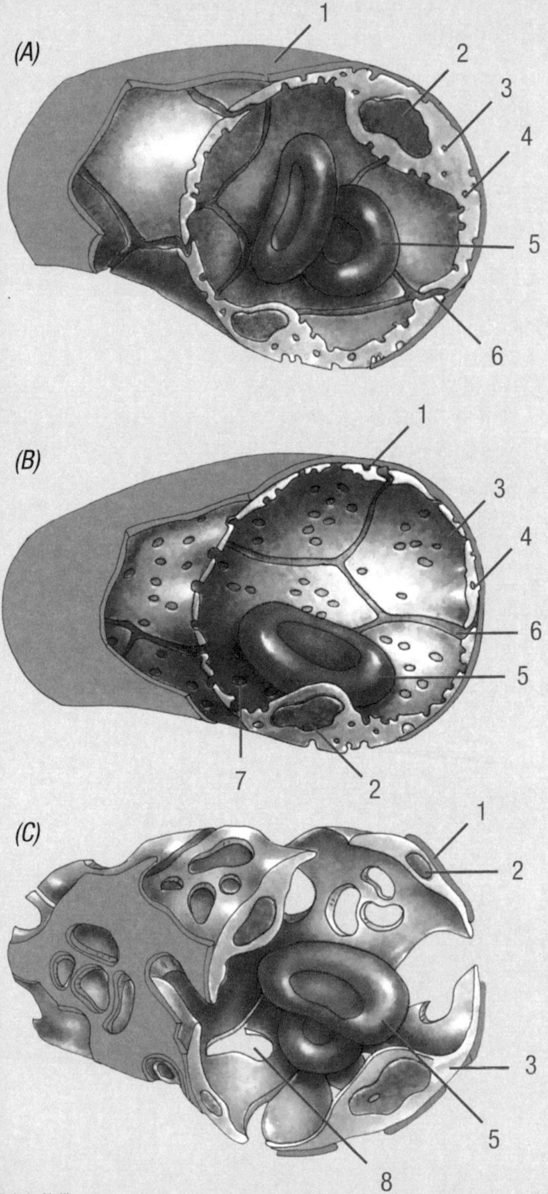
(A)
1
2
3
4
5
6
(B)
1
3
4
6
5
7
2
(C)
1
2
3
5
8

Lymphatics

Upper - lymphatic network showing interconnections b/n nodes & vessels

Middle - image of larger lymphatic vessels which drain to the LNs

Lower - network of lymphatics.

Guide - lymphatic drainage of the R & L sides of the body via the thoracic ducts.

Lymphatics form extensive networks b/n local LNs. Their vessels are thinner more numerous and have many valves. They mop up the excessive fluid and protein left behind from the capillary beds.

Only the larger vessels have any muscle or elasticity in their walls. There is an extensive and diverse network of superficial and deep vessels in all tissues.

If this is disrupted by disease or surgery the limb or region will swell up to 4X their original size.

1 lymph node (LN)

2 collecting lymphatic vessel

3 lymphatic capillaries draining into the collecting duct

4 adventitia layer – loose CT -collagen fibres

5 tunica media – CT, minimal elastic fibres, few muscle fibres

6 endothelium

7 valves

8 deep larger lymphatic network - fibres attached to tissue to improve draining with swelling

9 smaller superficial lymphatic capillaries

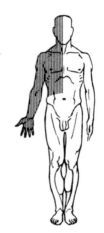

© A. L. Neill

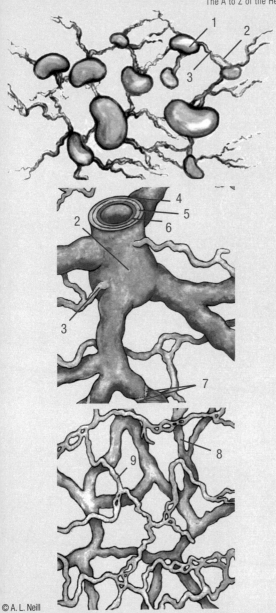

Lymphatic

Microscopic MP

The lymphatic vessel is thin walled, highly directed and branched. Endothelial cells open to allow fluid to flow in from the surrounding T but overlap with increased internal P to prevent the loss of the fluid, or its backflow. Lymphatics are opened by swollen T due to the anchoring filaments attached to the surrounding parenchyma.

1   lymphatic vessel
2   lymph
3   flow of the lymph -

> i = inflow through the open gaps of the endothelial cells
>
> t = will go through the closed valve
>
> b = stopped backflow by the closed valve

4   overlapping endothelial cells
5   lymphatic valve

> c = closed
>
> o = open

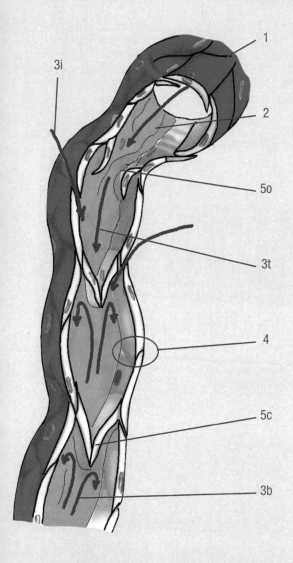

1

3i

2

5o

3t

4

5c

3b

Lymph node

Schema

Lymphatic vessels bring lymph into LN - one way flow - which moves through to the medulla. After leaving, the lymph may go to other LNs or to collecting ducts before draining to the venous system via either the R or L thoracic duct.

1 afferent lymphatic vessel (v= valves)

2 cortex

3 germinal centre

4 outer cells – exposed first to the lymph

5 cortical sinus

6 medulla

7 medullary sinus

8 hilus

9 efferent lymphatics (v = valves)

10 capsule

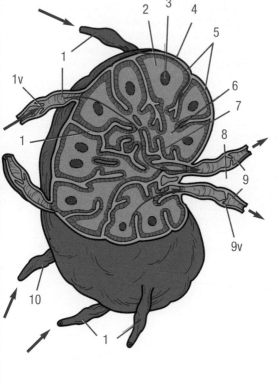

Veins

Microscopic MP
Large & medium veins have a similar structure.
They carry B to the heart.

They provide as little R to the BF as possible. Blood may be static in their lumens and they function as a "storage" for additional blood to return to the circulating system if needed, up to 500mls. Hence there are more veins than arteries. They have large very smooth lumens (5) to prevent clotting – lined by tightly connected endothelial cells (1) - THE TUNICA INTIMA, which may have semilunar valves in them partic. in the LL to facilitate venous return, while reducing R to flow. The smooth muscle layer is minimal with little or no elastic tissue partic in smaller veins - THE TUNICA MEDIA. Surrounding CT carries the BVs of the BVs, the vasa vasorum and N endings - the TUNICA EXTERNA or ADVENTITIA.

1 endothelium

2 BM

3 smooth muscle

4 CT containing fatty tissue / small BVs / Ns

5 lumen

6 valves

TUNICA INTIMA = 1+2+6

TUNICA MEDIA = 3

TUNICA EXTERNA = ADVENTITIA = 4

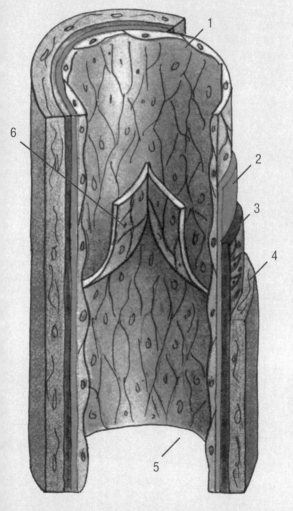

1

6

2

3

4

5

Cardiac muscle cells = CMCs = cardiac myocytes

Microscopic HP

These highly structured cells closely resemble skeletal muscle cells. Their contractile elements (9,10) are the same - thin attached actin filaments glide over the thick myosin filaments shortening the length and thickening the width of the muscle cell. Calcium ions are released deep into the cell via the transverse tubules (4) stimulating the large stores of calcium in the SR (5) to be released to maintain and deepen the intensity of the contraction and depolarization for longer than in the skeletal muscle cell - this can be further enhanced with Calcium channel blockers and this spreads rapidly from cell to cell via the gap junctions (7) - so the entire muscle tissue acts more as a unit than as single cells - functional syncytium. These branched cells contract in multiple planes.

1 nucleus
2 mitochondrium *(pl a)*
3 sarcolemma
4 transverse tubule (invagination from the sarcolemma)
5 sarcoplasmic reticulum (SR)
6 intercalated disc
7 gap junction
8 branched CMC
9 thick contractile filament = myosin
10 thin contractile filament = actin
11 contractile unit = sarcomere (Z band to Z band)
12 Z band for the attachment of the actin filaments

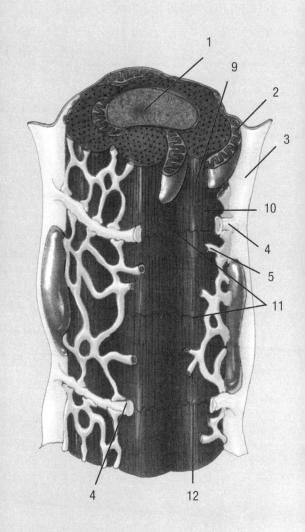

Cardiac muscle cells = CMCs = cardiac myocytes

Microscopic MP

These highly structured cells closely resemble skeletal muscle cells. Their contractile elements are the same as is their contractile unit – the sarcomere (11), although it is smaller. However they function more like smooth muscle cells in that they act as a syncytium with special devices for increasing conductivity b/n them ↑"leakiness" - gap junctions (7). They continually contract and relax in a cyclical fashion but have specific Ca^{2+} channels (4) and large Calcium ion stores (5) to ensure this is highly coordinated, and can be altered in intensity. Because of their branches (8) and tight intercellular connections - intercalalated discs (6), contraction can occur simultaneously and in multiple planes.

1   nucleus

2   mitochondrium *(pl a)*

3   sarcolemma

4   transverse tubule (invagination from the sarcolemma)

5   sarcoplasmic reticulum

6   intercalated disc

7   gap junction

8   branched CMC

9   thick contractile filament = myosin

10   thin contractile filament = actin

11   contractile unit = sarcomere (Z band to Z band)

12   Z band for the attachment of the actin filaments

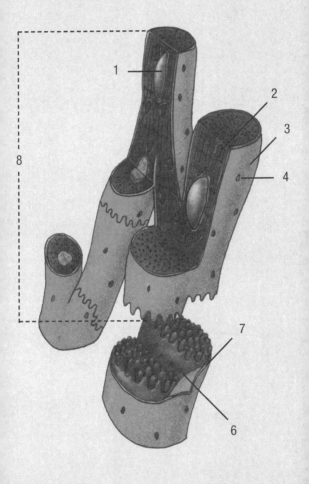

Myocardium - Cardiac muscle tissue

Macroscopic

Transverse view through the R and L ventricles.

The section through the ventricular walls demonstrates the difference in thickness of the R & L ventricles. This is due to their different and separate circulations – the RV pumps blood to the pulmonary system and the LV pumps blood to the rest of the body including to the heart itself a much higher pressured system – requiring more force to push the blood through it. Note the cavities of the ventricles are the same.*

1   post. interventricular artery + middle cardiac vein

2   visceral pericardium = epicardium

3   cavity of the LV

4   terminal cardiac artery

5   papillary muscle (if chordate tendini attached)

6   pericardial fat

7   ant. interventricular art. + great cardiac vein

8   endocardium – lining inside the heart cavities

9   cavity of the RV

10 interventricular septum

* the thickness of the ventricular walls is highly variable, it increases with age and with increased Peripheral resistance

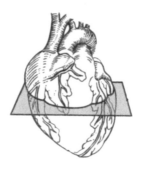

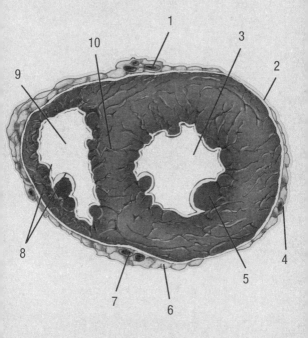

Heart – **development** up to 4 weeks

First   *lateral view of the embryo - 17 days*
Second   *developing heart pump from endothelial tubes 10-21 days*

The heart forms as 2 endothelial tubes which fuse and begin to pump spontaneously.

Angiogenic clusters form blood vessels around the yolk sac. The endothelial tubes continue from the "heart pump" and carry blood around the dorsum of the embryo, while the developing blood pools deliver the blood to the heart.

1 embryo
2 heart tube a = arterial end v = venous end
3 coalescing blood pools
4 angiogenic clusters
5 yolk sac
6 chorion
7 placenta
8 connecting stalk (later umbilicus)
9 amniotic sac
10 dorsal aorta
11 myotomes – future muscle
12 endocardial tubes
13 pericardial sac

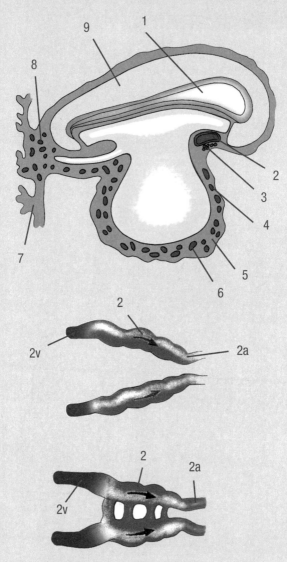

Heart – development up to 4 weeks *cont/*

Third fused heart tube from endothelial tubes 22-26 days
Fourth lateral view of the embryo – 22 -26 days
Fifth transverse view through the head of the embryo showing the dorsal
aortae and the endocardial tubes 20-24 days

The heart tube begins to pump spontaneously.

The angiogenic clusters coalesce into continuous channels forming blood vessels around the yolk sac, and then "vessels" to carry blood around the dorsum of the embryo, and then join with the "vessels" returning with nutrients to the heart.

1 embryo

2 heart tube a = arterial end v = venous end

3 coalescing blood pools

4 angiogenic clusters

5 yolk sac

6 chorion

7 placenta

8 connecting stalk (later umbilicus)

9 amniotic sac

10 dorsal aorta

11 myotomes – future muscle

12 endocardial tubes

13 pericardial sac

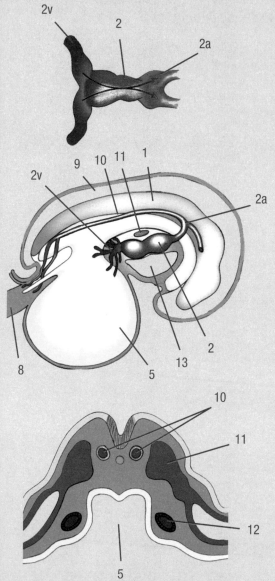

Heart – development 3 - 4weeks

Upper   ant. surface of dev heart with pericardial sac opened
Middle   heart tube beginning to fold
Lower   heart showing folding and dev of the 4 chambers

The heart tube pumps spontaneously and the circulation becomes a closed circuit. The tube forms swellings or chambers - and these chambers begin to curve on themselves forming the final 4 chambres.

Dorsal aortae leave the pericardial cavity and curve around the embryo.

1   1st aortic arch

2   bulbus cordis + future ventricles R&L

3   pericardial cavity

4   atria

5   sinus venosus - later vena cavae

6   dorsal aortae

7   truncus arteriosus

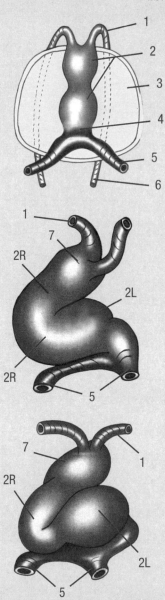

Heart – development 5 - 8 weeks

A - section
through truncus arteriosus to show the developing 2 circulatory systems

B - section
through atria & ventricles to show the developing 4 chambered heart

1   truncus arterosus – future arterial trunks

2   future atrial chambers L & R

3   future ventricular chambers L & R

4   future caval system of venous return

5   truncoconal swellings – develops into 11

6   endocardial cushions – develops into 12f

7   muscular interventricular septum – develops into 12m

8   atrioventricular canal L & R

9   aortic outflow

10 pulmonary trunk outflow

11 aortico-pulmonary septum

12 interventricular septum –

f= fibrous/membranous m = muscular parts

13 septum & ostium primum

14 septum & ostium secundu

15 papillary muscles

16 chordae tendineae

17 valve for coronary sinus

18 valve for IVC

19 cristae terminalis

20 SVC inflow in LA

21 L atrium -
    inflow of pulmonary arteries

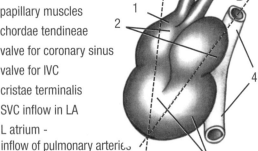

© A. L. Neill

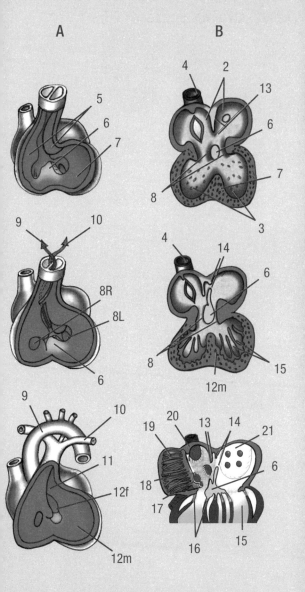

A

B

Heart - external surfaces

Anterior

1. L carotid artery
2. L subclavian artery
3. ligamentum arteriosum
4. L pulmonary artery
5. pericardium
6. L auricle
7. L coronary artery
   a = ant. interventricular branch
   c = circumflex branch
8. great cardiac vein
9. LV
10. RV
11. IVC
12. small cardiac vein
13. RA
14. R coronary artery
15. R auricle
16. SVC
17. R brachiocephalic trunk

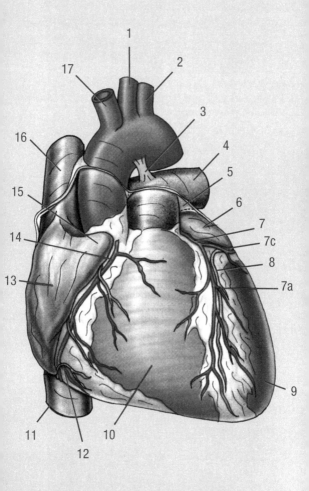

Pericardium

Layers around the heart - lateral view
Mid sagittal view - heart in the mediastinum

The heart sits inside a double layered bag the pericardium. One layer is adherent to the heart surface, supports the coronary vessels and extends to the roots of the great vessels – visceral pericardium (3) this then doubles back leaving a space (4) filled with a small amount of pericardial fluid (15mls) and forms the outer parietal layer (5) which fuses with the strong outer fibrous layer (1). This fixes the capsule to the fibrous central tendon of the diaphragm (2).

1   fibrous pericardium

2   central tendon of the diaphragm

3   visceral pericardium

4   pericardial space – site of the cardiac sinuses

5   parietal pericardium

6   R ventricle

7   R atrium

8   diaphragm muscle

9   endocardium – inner lining of the heart chambers continuous with ...

10 endothelium – inner lining of the BVs

11 aorta

12 mediastium

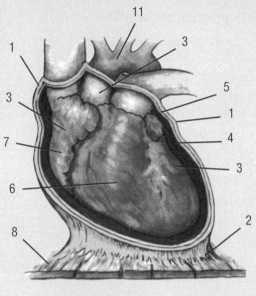

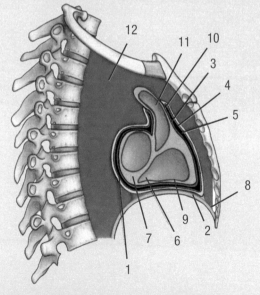

Heart - external surfaces

Diaphragmatic surface = base of heart
"Posterior"

1 SVC
2 pulmonary veins L= left / R= right
3 RA
4 marginal branch of R coronary artery
5 RV
6 middle cardiac vein
7 post. Interventricular artery
8 LV
9 coronary sinus
10 LA
11 pulmonary arteries L = left / R = right

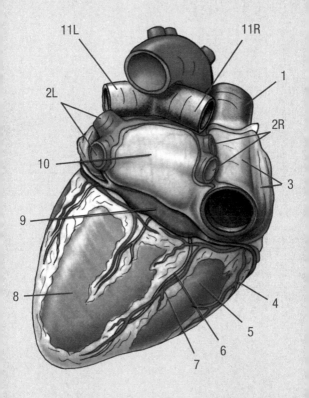

Pericardial sinuses

Anterior view – heart removed
The heart is encased in a double layered sac – the pericardium.

The adherent or visceral layer reflects in areas to form the outer or parietal layer forming sinuses – or areas where the heart can be separated from the cavity.

The heart sits in the mediastinum on the central ligament of the diaphragm.

1 aorta
   a = ascending / r = arch / t = thoracic

2 pulmonary trunk

3 pulmonary veins
   L = left / R = right

4 sinuses
   o = oblique / t = transverse

5 diaphragm – central tendon

6 Vena cava
   i = IVC / s = SVC

7 pulmonary arteries
   L = left / R = right

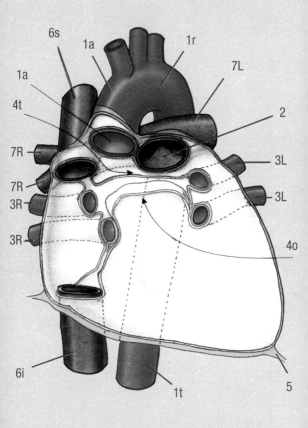

6s

1a

1r

7L

1a

4t

2

7R

3L

7R

3L

3R

3R

4o

6i

5

1t

Surface projection of the Heart
Auscultation of Heart sounds

Anterior Chest

The Heart is covered and protected by the Sternum = breast bone and rib cage, hence heart sounds indicating valve closures cannot be heard directly over the valves but to the transmitted areas in the surrounding spaces. There are 2 main HS - S1 associated with AV valve closure and S2 associated with aortic & pulmonary valve closure.

Diagram shows the site of the valves and the site of best auscultation. Splitting of S1 & S2 indicate gaps in the closures of the valves which is often a sign of pathology.

1	pulmonary	RV ➡ pulm. trunk	L 2nd ICS	S2
2	aortic	LV ➡ aorta	R 2nd ICS	S2
3	bicuspid mitral	LA ➡ LV	L 5th ICS parasternal edge	S1
4	tricuspid	RA ➡ RV	L 5th ICS parasternal edge	S1
5	apex beat		L 5th ICS nipple line = midclavicular line	
6	Sternum			
7	Manubrium			
8	Jugular notch			

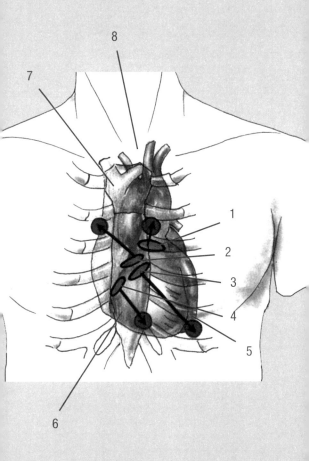

Left Atrium

Posterolateral view - wall of the LA sectioned and reflected

The LA receives B from the pulmonary veins all 4 emptying into the cavity and admits B to the LV, where it goes to the systemic circulation. In the foetal circulation B also comes from the RA and is prevented from returning via the valve which seals in the first months of birth separating the 2 circulations – if it does not the person is said to have a "hole" in their heart.

1　pulmonary veins

2　"valve" of fossa ovale

3　LA

4　mitral valve = bicuspid valve

5　coronary sinus

6　LV

7　chordae tendini

8　auricle of LA

9　pulmonary trunk

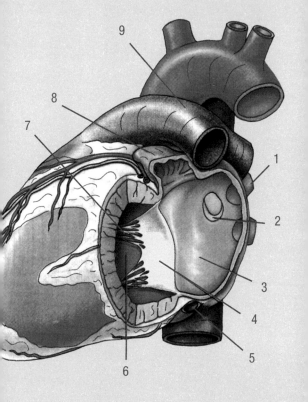

Right Atrium

view - wall of the RA sectioned and reflected

The RA receives B from the Vena Cavae and admits it to the RV, where it goes to the pulmonary circulation. In the foetal circulation this path is circumvented and the B goes from the RA to the LA via the foramen ovale - a hole in the interatrial septum. This is closed at birth and becomes fossa ovalis.

1. auricle of RA
2. ant. interventricular+ great cardiac vein
3. apex of the heart + RV
4. R coronary art
5. tricuspid valve
6. cardiac sinus o= opening / v = valve
7. IVC + valve of IVC
8. fossa ovalis + limbus of fossa (8L)
9. musculi pectinati
10. crista terminalis

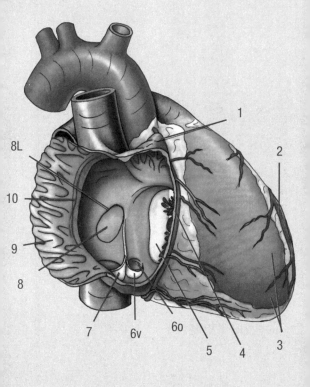

8L

10

9

8

7   6v   6o

5   4   3

1

2

Conduction in the Heart

Coronal view of the heart – anterior outer wall removed

Each HB is a coordinated contraction and relaxation of the myocardium - the cardiac cycle - facilitated by the conducting system which begins in the SA node in the RA radiates across the atria before going to the AV node to reach the ventricles. Contraction begins at the base of the ventricles due to the conduction of the depolarization stimulus via the Purkinje fibres - a series of insulated specialized cardiac cells.

1 aortic arch

2 aortic sinus

3 sinoatrial node (SA)

4 RA

5 atrioventricular node (AV)

6 bundle of His

7 IVC

8 Purkinje fibres inserted into myocardium of the ventricular wall

9 R & L bundle branches of Purkinje fibres

10 wall of LV

11 papillary muscles

12 chordea tendineae = fibres to connect AV valves to the ventricle wall

13 internodal pathways

14 pulmonary trunk

15 conduction barrier b/n atria & ventricles

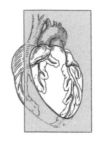

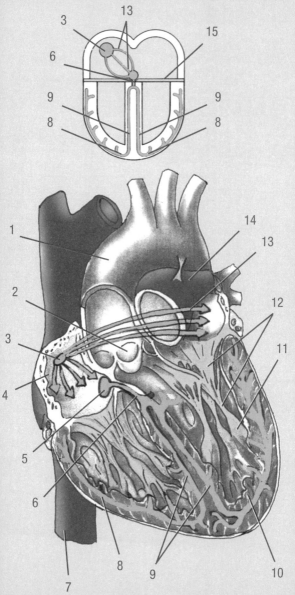

© A. L. Neill

Heart - internal structure

Anterior view –
slice through in a coronal plane to see all 4 chambres

1 aortic arch

2 L pulmonary arteries

3 L pulmonary veins

4 LA

5 mitral valve = bicuspid valve

6 aortic valve – semilunar cusps

7 papillary muscles

8 interventricular septum

9 R ventricular wall

10 chordae tendineae (attached to 7)

11 tricupsid valve

12 IVC

13 RA

14 pulmonary valve

15 pulmonary trunk arterial

16 SVC

17 ligamentum arteriosum

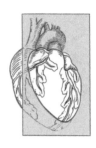

© A. L. Neill

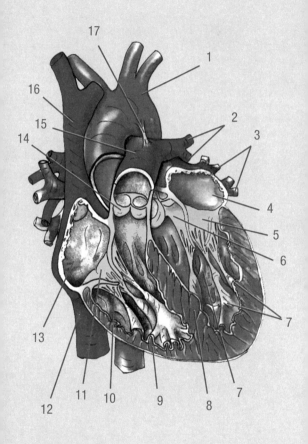

Fibrous Skeleton of the Heart = Tendon of the heart

Transverse plane - Superior view
Atria removed

A = anterior P = posterior

Interconnected collagen fibres + fibrocartilage rings & septa make up the fibrous skeleton of the heart. It joins all valves, extends to the pulmonary & aortic trunks, the septa of the heart and forms the chordae tendineae. Atria and ventricles are isolated electrically via the skeleton which transmits and insulates the Purkinje fibre bundles. The myocardium embeds into the skeleton, which acts as a tendon.

1 pulmonary fibrous ring

2 conus tendon = fibres connecting 1+4

3 roof of conus arteriosus

4 aortic fibrous ring

5 R AV fibrous ring

6 tricuspid valve

7 R fibrous trigone = fibres connecting 4+5+8

8 L AV fibrous ring

9 mitral valve

10 L fibrous trigone = fibres connecting 4+8

11 aortic valve

12 pulmonary valve

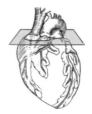

A

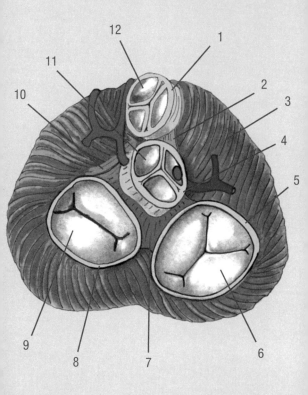

P

Heart Valves

Transverse plane - Superior view
Atria removed - coronary vessels left intact
Upper - pulmonary and aortic valves closed
Lower – bicuspid and tricuspid valves closed

A = anterior P = posterior

1 Pulmonary valve (transmits B from
   RV→ pulmonary trunk)
   has 3 semi-lunar* valves ant., R& L

2 Aortic valve (transmits blood from LV aorta)
   Thas 3 semi-lunar* valves R, L & post.

3 bicuspid valve = mitral valve (transmits B
   from LA→LV) and is part of the fibrous skeleton of the
   heart – attached to the endocardium via papillary
   muscles, fibrous strands and has 2 valves ant. & post.

4 tricuspid valve (transmits B from RA→RV) and is part of
   the fibrous skeleton of the heart – attached to the
   endocardium via papillary muscles and fibrous strands
   and has 3 valves ant. & post. + septal

5 fibrous skeleton, a continuous fibrous +
   fibocartilagenous structure connecting: the valves,
   muscle layers, septa and arterial trunks

6 L coronary artery
   a- ant. interventricular artery
   c- circumflex art

7 R coronary artery
   o- opening into the aortic sinus
   p- post. interventricular artery

8 chordae tendineae fibrous strands of collagen connecting
   the valve flaps to the endocardium

9 valve cusps - flaps of endothelial lined CT

similar to the venous valves in structure

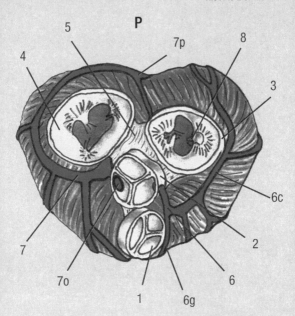

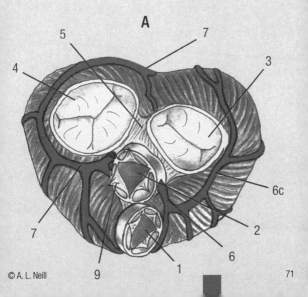

© A. L. Neill

Left Ventricle

Heart uplifted and rotated to the R so that the posterior surface is in front exposing the L ventricle - wall removed to show the interior of the LV

The L V pumps B → the aorta via the infundibulum (funnel) through the aortic valve into the aortic sinus (or swelling). The 2 coronary arteries arise from the aortic sinus.

Hence oxygenated B leaves the L V to supply the rest of the body. This is a high P system with a lot of peripheral resistance (PR) The pressures needed to overcome this PR determine a person's BP - the systolic (highest) and diastolic (lowest) Ps.

1 chordae tendineae

2 aortic valve

3 infundibulum

4 papillary muscles
  a = ant / p = post.

5 apex of the heart

6 trabeculae = trabeculae carneae

7 mitral valve
  a = ant / p = post. cusps

8 circumflex coronary art. → post interventricular art

9 LA

10 coronary sinus

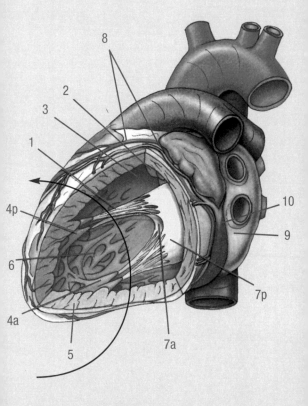

Right Ventricle

Anterior view – anterior wall removed

The R V pumps B → the pulmonary trunk through the pulmonary valve and supplies the ↓P pulmonary circulation. Hence deoxygenated B leaves this ventricle to become oxygenated in the lungs.

The myocardium does not have a lot of R and therefore pumping is relatively easy, hence the R V wall is thin ~ ½ to ⅓ the thickness of the L V wall.

It receives B from the systemic circulation making it vulnerable to infections and disease particularly on the valves, the result often being valvular disease ± P changes ± R sided failure.

1 ligamentum arteriosum
2 pulmonary valve
3 conus arteriosus
4 papillary muscles
   a = ant / p = post. / s = septal
5 apex of the heart
6 trabeculae = trabeculae carneae
7 tricuspid valve
8 R coronary artery
9 RA
10 SVC

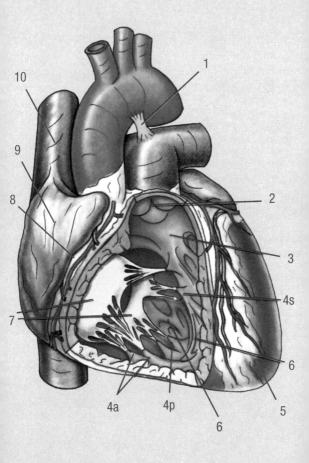

Mediastinum

Definition - the thoracic space b/n the lungs

It is further subdivided into 4 components:

1 *superior* – above the heart to the root of the neck

2 *anterior* – in front of the heart

3 *middle* – the cavity for the heart

4 *posterior* – the space behind the heart inferior border the diaphragm

5 mediastinum = 1 + 2 +3 + 4

6 apex of the lung (above the ribs)

7 L & R lung

8 roots of the lung L & R (opening in the pleura for the pulmonary trunks)

9 pleura for the lungs

10 central tendon of the diaphragm

11 muscular crura of the diaphragm – opening for the oesophagus

12 arcuate ligament – opening for the aorta

13 pleural space below the lungs

14 opening in the central tendon for the IVC

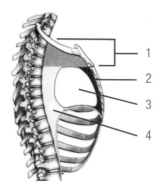

© A. L. Neill

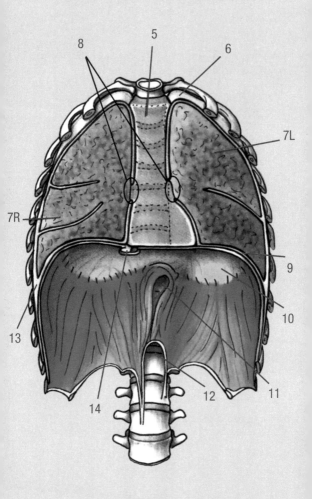

Mediastinum + Pleural Cavities = Thoracic cavity

Anterior – coronal plane

The space b/n the root of the neck and the diaphragm is the thoracic cavity made up of the 2 pleural cavities containing the R & L lungs, and the mediastinum containing the heart, roots of the great vessels, oesophagus and trachea. A framework of muscles surrounds this space supporting the ribs, upper limbs, shoulders and back.

1 thyroid

2 thyroidea ima

3 pleural lining parietal

4 pulmonary arteries L

5 heart borders R & L note the borders are wider than the Sternum - (not shown)

6 lung surface with adherent visceral pleural layer

7 pleural cavity beyond the lung mass

8 apex of heart

9 base of heart on the central tendon of the diaphragm

10 adjacent/adherent pleural and pericardial linings

11 apex of the lung - note is outside the thoracic cavity

12 jugular veins & carotid arteries

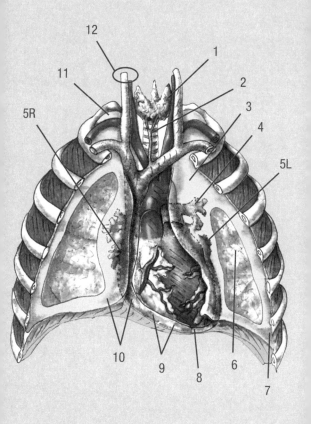

Mediastinum + Pleural Cavities = Thoracic cavity

Transverse – A-anterior / P-posterior

The space b/n the root of the neck and the diaphragm is the thoracic cavity made up of the 2 pleural cavities containing the R & L lungs, and the mediastinum containing the heart, roots of the great vessels, oesophagus and trachea. A framework of muscles surrounds this space supporting the ribs, upper limbs, shoulders and back.

1 heart
2 lungs R & L
3 oesophagus
4 aorta (descending)
5 trachea
6 T6
7 SC
8 pleural lining
9 pericardium

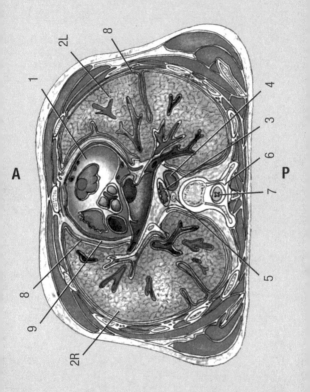

2L

8

1

4

3

6

7

5

A

P

8

9

2R

Mediastinum lateral view

looking into cavity from the L

The aorta ascends and then turns to descend from the L - the L recurrent laryngeal N curves around it before ascending to the larynx. Hemiazygous and accessory azygos veins seen from this side.

1. trachea
2. aortic arch
3. brachiocephalic trunk
4. thymus
5. pulmonary arteries
6. phrenic N
7. atria
8. dome of diaphragm
9. oesophageal plexus

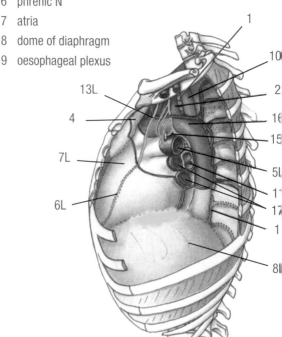

© A. L. Neil

Mediastinum lateral view

looking into cavity from the R

The heart points to the L with the SVC - RA- IVC in a line from superior to inferior (IVC outside the mediastinum). The oesophagus and azygos veins can be seen from this side, note the close association b/n the oesophageal plexus and the R vagus N on the heart.*

10 oesophagus

11 main bronchus

12 azygous

13 vagus N

14 IC NV bundle

15 recurrent laryngeal N

16 aorta

17 pulmonary veins

18 hemiazygous

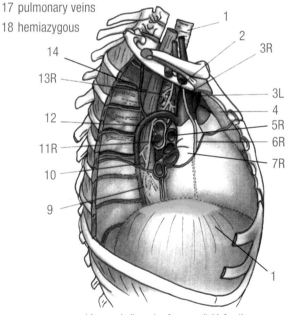

** hence similar pain of myocardial infarction
and acid reflux (heart attack and indigestion)*

Superior Mediastinum =
Roots of the great vessels

Anterior view
Boundaries of the superior mediastinum are:

Anterior – Manubrium
Inferior – sternal angle to inferior border of T4
Laterally – parietal pleura of the lungs
Posterior – T1-4
Superior – jugular notch to superior border of T1

1. L common carotid art
2. L internal jugular vein
3. L subclavian art.
4. L subclavian vein
5. L brachiocephalic vein
6. arch of the aorta
7. Manubrium
8. L pulmonary art
9. L main bronchus
10. pulmonary trunk
11. Sternum
12. descending aorta
13. SVC outside the manubriosternal border
14. R pulmonary art
15. L brachiocephalic vein
16. Rib 2
17. R subclavian vein
18. Clavicle
19. R subclavian artery
20. Rib 1
21. R internal jugular vein
22. R common carotid art
23. trachea
24. oesophagus

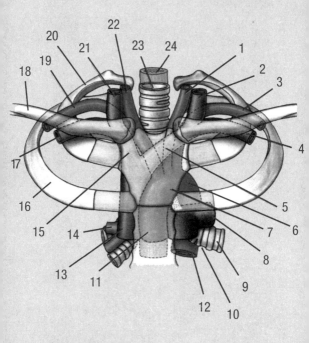

Blood supply of the Adrenal Glands AKA Suprarenal gland and the Renal aas

A Anterior view of the posterior abdominal wall demonstrating relationship b/n the kidneys & the diaphragm; showing adrenal artery origin from the abdominal aorta

B Anterior view of the adrenal & renal arterial aas showing adrenal supply from the inf. phrenic a

The adrenals sit on top of the kidneys and share their BS via aas & in 1/3 of cases as a branch of the renal artery. In the other 2/3 of cases the adrenal artery is a branch of the inferior phrenic artery & the abdominal aorta directly. The outer arteries of the renal bed form a vascular ring (AKA exorenal arcade), anatomizing with the gonadal arteries, the adrenal arteries and the renal & ureteric arteries. The R & L glands may have different & multiple origins. The R adrenal gland is generally lower than the L because of the liver. The veins drain to the IVC.

1   opening in the diaphragm for the oesophagus
2   inferior phrenic a
3   superior adrenal a
4   diaphragm
5   inferior adrenal a
6   kidney
7   adrenal & renal veins
8   abdominal aorta
9   IVC
10 adrenal gland
11 exorenal arcade supplies the surrounding adipose T & the renal capsule
12 ureter & ureteric a
13 middle adrenal a
14 renal a
15 inferior mesenteric a
16 gonadal a (♀ ovarian / ♂ testicular)
17 superior mesenteric a
18 coeliac trunk

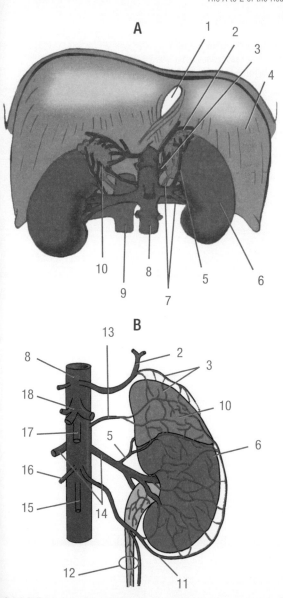

Blood supply of the Alveoli

The BS of the alveoli forms the R circulation of the Heart. It is the area of O_2 / CO_2 exchange, as well as the respiratory acid / base balance. B/n the RBCs and the "air" is a thin bm and the thin walls of 2 cells the endothelium lining the respiratory capillaries and the cells lining the internal surface of the alveoli. The capillaries are dilated to provide maximum surface area for gas exchange.

The arterioles bring deoxygenated B to the alveoli;

The capillaries are the site of oxygenation & the venules take oxygenated B back to the heart.

1   bronchiole
2   alveolar capillary bed
3   venule
4   alveoli
5   arteriole

B
C
D
E
F
G
H
I
J
K
L
M
N
O
P
Q
R
S
T
U
V
W
X
Y
Z

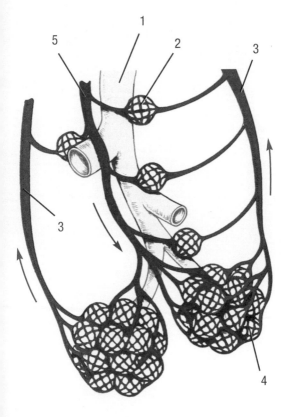

© A. L. Neill

Blood supply of the Anus & Rectum - Arterial

Description: The arterial supply of the rectum and anal canal like the facial vessels is richly anastomotic – particularly at the ano-rectal junction.

1 Aorta

2 L colic a

3 Sigmoid a

4 Ext. iliac a

5 Int. iliac a

6 Pudendal a

7 Anal canal + recto arterial plexus & anastomoses

8 Pelvic diaphragm

9 Inf. rectal a

10 Middle rectal a

11 Rectum

12 Superior rectal a

13 Inf mesenteric a

14 IVC

© A. L. Neill

Blood supply of the Anus & Rectum - Lymphatic

Description: The lymphatic drainage of the rectum and anal canal is intimately related to the pelvic and inguinal lymphatic drainage. Infections &/or neoplasms in these areas spread rapidly because of this highly branched and interconnected network.

1　Aorta + Para-aortic LNs (= Lateral aortic LNs)

2　Inf mesenteric a

3　Sigmoid a

4　Middle rectal art. + rectal LNs

5　Int. iliac art. + iliac LNs

6　Pudenal art. + LNs

7　Pelvic diaphragm

8　LNs connecting to the superficial inguinal LN networks

9　Inf. rectal LNs

10　Coccygeal LNs – post. to the Rectum

11　Sacral LNs – post. to the Rectum

12　Rectum + Para-rectal LNs

13　Superior rectal a + superior rectal LNs

14　Common iliac LNs – medial, lateral & subaortic

© A. L. Neill

Blood supply of the Anus & Rectum - Venous

Description: The venous supply of the rectum and anus is particularly important. It is one of the sites where the LP - low resistance portal venous system meets the HP - high resistance systemic circulation. Any build up of pressure in the portal system will result in the ballooning and expansion of the thin-walled portal veins. This results in Hemorrhoids, which form along the dentate line and may protrude through the anal opening.

1 brs from the SI to the Superior Mesenteric V
2 R Colic V
3 Common Iliac V
   3e – external iliac V
   3i - internal iliac V
4 Sigmoid V
5 Rectal veins
   5i – inferior rectal V
   5m – middle rectal V
   5s - superior rectal V
6 Internal pudendal V
7 Pelvic Diaphragm
8 Anal canal
9 Recto-venous plexus = Porto-venous anastomosis
10 Rectum
11 IVC

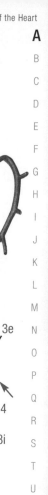

11

1

2

3

3e

5s

4

10

5m

3i

6

9

7

5i

8

© A. L. Neill

Blood supply of the Appendix & Ileocaecal junction - Arterial supply

wall cut away from the LI, caecum to show relationships

mesentery removed from around the BVs which travel in this – separate appendicular mesentery for its BV

1 mesentery (cut)
2 ileum
3 straight arteries = arteriae rectae
4 arterial arcades
5 appendicular art.
6 appendix v = appendix orifice
7 ileocolic art.
   brs –
   a = ant. caecal art.
   c = colic
   i = ileal
   p = post. caecal art.
8 lymphatic follicules = Peyers' patches
9 ascending colon

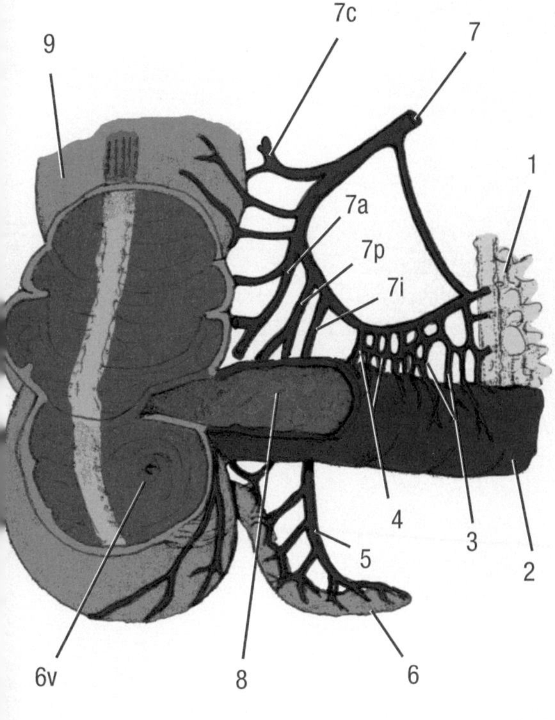
7c
7
9
1
7a
7p
7i
4
3
5
2
6v
8
6

Blood supply of the Arm
- Arterial supply

Anterior view

1   aortic arch
2   R brachiocephalic art
3   subclavian art
4   axillary art
5   brachial art
6   radial art
7   ulnar art
8   superfical palmar arch
9   deep palmar arch
10 common palmar digital art
11 digital art (proper)

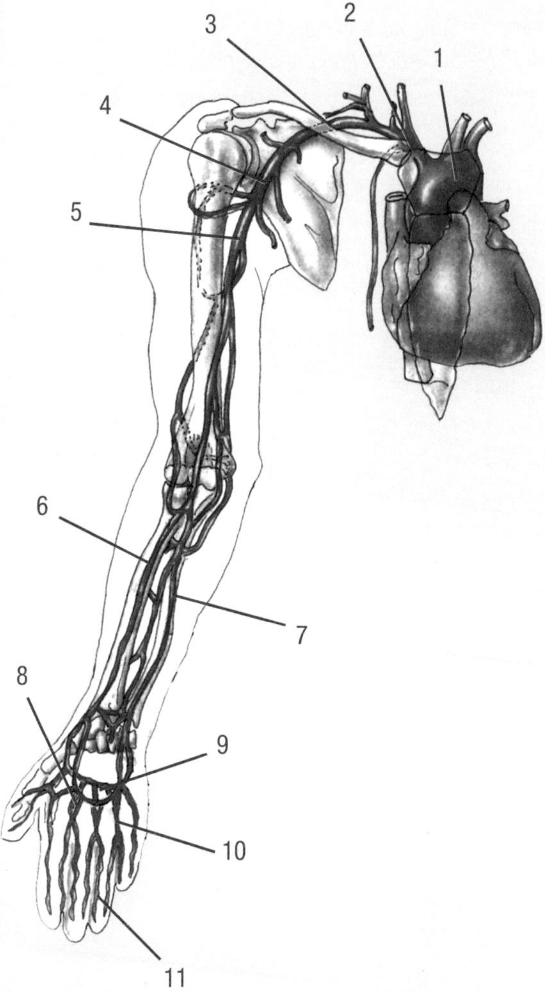
1
2
3
4
5
6
7
8
9
10
11

Blood Supply of the Arm

- Venous supply

Anterior - Superficial veins
Anterior – Superficial and deep veins

As with the LL, the arm or UL has 2 venous systems – the superficial accessed clinically for most B sampling. The supf veins lie outside the deep fascia and do not have an arterial equivalent - the deep veins follow the arteries generally deep to the deep fascia.

Purple vessels represent the deep system.

1 subclavian vein

2 acromial br

3 cephalic vein

4 axillary vein

5 cutaneous axillary vein

6 basilic vein

7 median cubital vein

8 median vein

9 palmar venous plexus

10 circumflex

11 subscapular veins

12 brachial veins (profunda brachii)

13 ulnar veins

14 radial veins

15 interosseous veins

16 palmar arches supf & deep

17 metacarpal veins

18 proper palmar digital veins

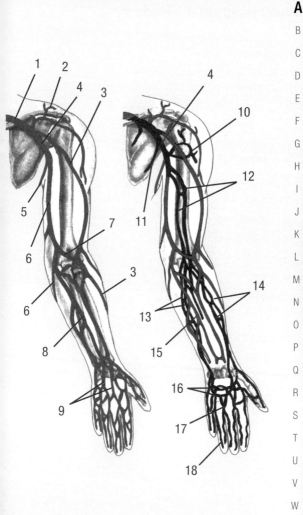

© A. L. Neill

Blood supply of the Bladder

Macroscopic view
Lateral - male - BS

The bladder is a collapsible bag which has a copious anastomotic BS intimately related to the adjacent structures - prostate in the male - vagina and uterus in the female.

1   int. iliac a & v
2   obliterated umbilical a
3   superior vesical a
4   fundus
5   median umbilical lig
6   vesical venous plexus
7   prostate brs from inf. vesical a & v
8   prostate
9   urethra
10 seminal vesicles
11 middle rectal v
12 ductus deferens + a
13 ureter + uteric a + v
14 inf. vesical uteric a & v
15 inf. gluteal a & v

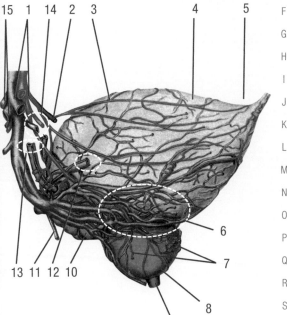

Blood supply of Bone - Arterial supply

Micro Schema

Most LBs have an outer compact bone shell and inner spongy bone which is thin in the bone shaft – diaphysis but present throughout the ends – epiphyses.

The central core is BM. This schema shows a cross section through the shaft of a LB.

1   outer lamellar circumferential system

2   osteon = Haversian system

3   cement line – b/n osteons – calcified GS

4   central BV

5   collagen fibres – helical with alternate directional turns in each layer of the osteon

6   inner lamellar circumferential system

7   spicule of spongy bone = trabecular bone = cancellous bone

8   spicules connect with each other along the force lines of the bone

9   BM

10 endosteum – lines inner bone surfaces – contains OG cells

11 BVs + central canal of the osteon

12 OC

13 Volkmann's canal – perforating osteon lamellae

14 periosteal space + inner periosteal layer

15 Sharpey's fibres – collagen fibres connecting to the bone T

16 periosteum – containing BS to the bone

17 interstitial lamellar bone – remnants of old remodelled osteons

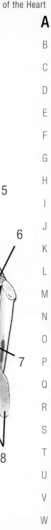

© A. L. Neill

Blood supply Brain & Spinal Cord overview
Brain

Schema of the brain – coronal

1 Skull = bony covering

2 meningeal vein

3 DM around the venous sinuses + communicating vessel

4 external cerebral vein

5 brain – nervous tissue

6 choroid plexus

7 deep cerebral vein

8 extracranial vein

9 extracranial art

10 meningeal art

11 superficial cerebral art

Spinal Cord

Schema of the SC – transverse

1 posterior spinal art

2 radicular branches a = anterior / L = lateral / p = posterior

3 arterial vasocorona

4 lateral artery

5 anterior radicular artery

6 branches of the superficial arterial network

7 anterior spinal artery

8 sucal art = ant. spinal art. (lies in the sulcus of the SC)

9 marginal zone (of Lissauer)

10 anterior horn = ventral motor horn

11 deep spinal art

12 substantia gelatinosa

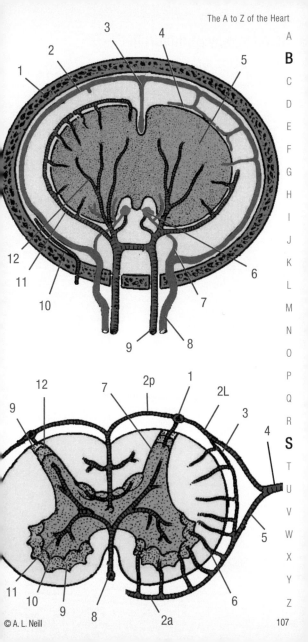

© A. L. Neill

Blood supply of the Brain

Inferior view – *Arterial supply*

The brain cannot be deprived of arterial blood for longer than 1 minute. The circle of Willis is the core of the BS from which the main arteries originate.

1 anterior spinal art.
2 vertebral art. – paired
3 post. inf. cerebellar art.
4 ant. inf. cerebellar art.
5 basilar artery – from the fusion of the paired vertebral arteries
6 pontine branches
7 post. cerebral art.
8 Circle of Willis = arterial circle ,
9 middle cerebral art
10 ant. cerebral art.
11 cerebellar arteries

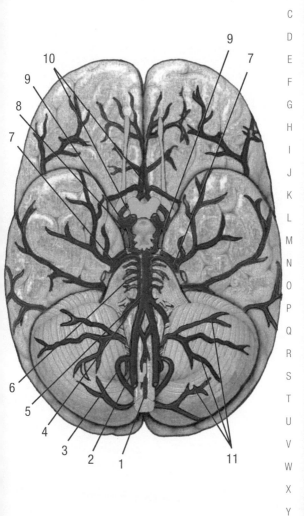

Blood supply of the Brain

Lateral view – venous drainage

On the surface of the brain there are many BVs which drain into a series of sinuses - endothelial lined channels b/n the 2 layers of the DM. They anastomose extensively and have no valves relying on gravity, cranial pressure and head movements for drainage. Superficial vessels drain to the superior sagittal sinus (1s) and deeper vessels drain to the straight sinus (4). The eyeball and facial areas drain to the cavernous sinus (8) and may bring infection into the cranial cavity.

1 sagittal sinus i = inferior / s = superior
2 connecting anastomosing veins
3 deep posterior cerebral veins
4 straight sinus
5 transverse sinus
6 sigmoid sinus (s-shaped)
7 petrosal sinus i =inferior / s = superior
8 cavernous sinus
9 internal jugular vein

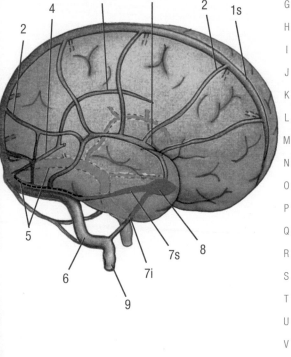

Blood supply of the Brainstem

Lateral view – arteries only

1 pontine cerebral art.

2 inferior colliculus

3 cerebral aqueduct

4 inferior quadrigeminal art.

5 superior vermis of cerebellum

6 superior cerebellar art.

7 dentate gyrus

8 anterior inferior cerebellar art.

9 cerebellar flocculus and nodulus

10 4th ventricle

11 posterior inferior cerebellar art.

12 central canal

13 posterior spinal art.

14 vertebral art. (paired vessels)

15 anterior spinal art.

16 paramedian art.

17 cuneate and gracile nuclei

18 inferior olivary nuclei

19 pons

20 basilar art (unpaired – fusion of the vertebrals)

21 posterior communicating art. (part of the circle of Willis)

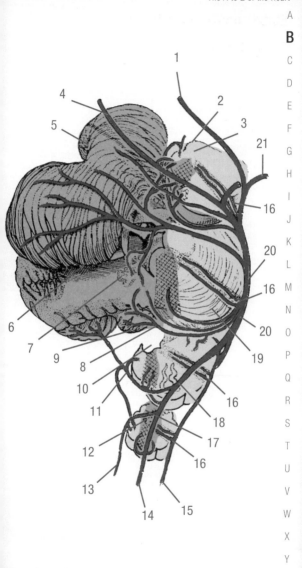

© A. L. Neill

Blood supply of the Breast

Anterior view - arterial supply

1 thoracoacromial a
2 pectoral br
3 lateral thoracic a
4 subscapular a
5 posterior intercostal a
6 perforating br
7 lateral mammary br
8 thoracodorsal a
9 internal thoracic a

  a = anterior intercostal br
  m = medial mammary br
  p = perforating br

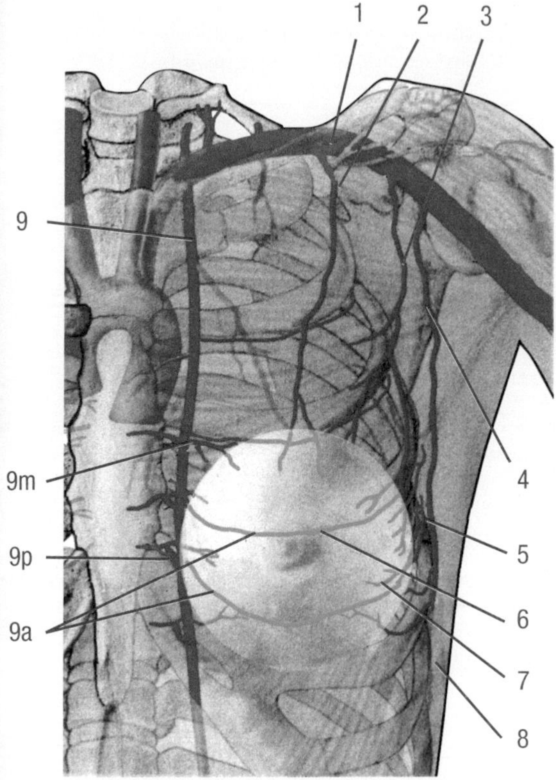
1
2
3
9
9m
9p
9a
4
5
6
7
8

Blood supply of the Breast

Anterior view - arterial supply and lymphatic drainage

The BS of the breasts are intimately related to their lymphatic drainage. There is a rich aas in the BS and the chest and axilla as well as BVs and lymphatic vessels which will cross over to the other breast. Hence spread of disease can occur b/n 1 breast and the other.

1 subclavian LNs

2 central axillary LNs

3 lateral axillary LNs

4 subclavian artery

5 deep axillary LNs

6 subscapular LNs

7 thoracic artery with lateral intercostal arteries

8 pectoral LNs

9 L internal mammary = anterior thoracic art

10 br b/n the R & L internal mammary arteries

11 anterior intercostal arteries*

12 L parasternal LNs – aa with the R nodes

13 ant chest wall – pectoral major

* *note there is an aa b/n the ant. & lat. IC art.*

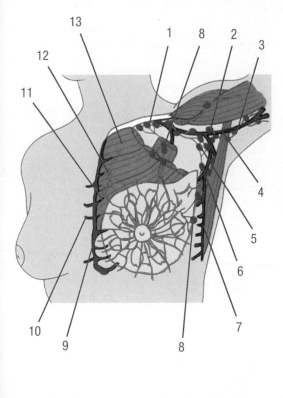

Blood supply of the Breast

Anterior view - Lymph Nodes and Venous drainage

The breast drains mainly to the 40 axillary LNs from 3 levels. Using Pectoralis Minor m as a guide these can be described as those lateral to Pec. Minor (3, 4, 6 & 9), medial to Pec. Minor (15 &18) & below Pec Minor (2 & 16), but the only palpable LNs are : the anterior & central LNs in the axilla and the supraclavicular LNs.

The venous supply mirrors the arterial supply and LNs flank the veins.

In breast cancer the number of axillary LNs involved is correlated to the number of axillary LNs involved - in both male & females, with particularly poor survival associated with supraclavicular LN involvement.

1   axillary v
2   central LNs
3   lateral LNs AKA Humeral LNs
4   subscapular LNs
5   subscapular v
6   pectoral LNs (Sorguis' LN)
7   lateral thoracic v
8   thoracodorsal v
9   paramammary LNs
10 superior lat quadrant
11 inferior lat quadrant
12 inferior medial quadrant
13 internal thoracic v
14 superior medial quadrant
15 parasternal LNs
16 interpectoral LNs (Rotter's LNs)
17 Pectoralis minor m
18 apical LNs
19 supraclavicular LNs (Virchow's LNs)

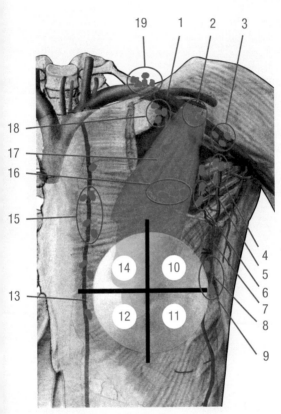

© A. L. Neill

Blood supply of the Cerebrum

Arterial supply
Inferior view
Lateral view
Sagittal view

The arteries supplying the cerebrum consist of 3 paired branches arising from the arterial circle or Circle of Willis: the anterior, middle and posterior cerebral arteries.

Their supply corresponds roughly although not absolutely with the cerebral lobes.

The brain is very sensitive to any deprivation of oxygen and will die if deprived for oxygen completely for longer than 1 min in normal circumstances.

A = cerebral tissue supplied by the ant. cerebral art. and its branches

M = cerebral tissue supplied by the middle cerebral art. and its branches

P = cerebral tissue supplied by the post. cerebral artery and its branches

1   anterior cerebral artery b = branches

2   anterior communicating artery

3   middle cerebral artery b = branches

4   posterior cerebral artery b = branches /
    c = calcarine branch / o = occipital branch

5   brainstem

6   corpus callosum g = genu / s = splenium

7   anterior perforating substance

8   thalamus

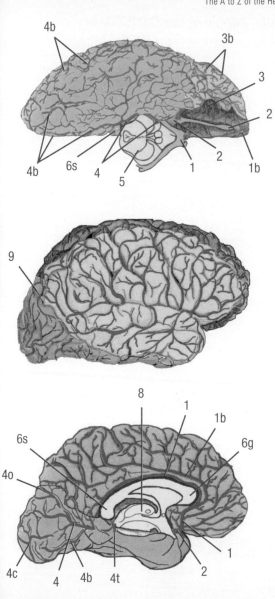

© A. L. Neill

Blood supply of the Cubital fossa
Deep structures - arterial supply

Anterior – skin, superficial and deep fascia removed
*   – superficial muscles divided*

1 biceps (cut) m = muscle t = tendon

2 musculocutaneous N

3 brachial art.

4 median N

5 ulnar art.

6 pronator teres m

7 radial art.

8 supinator m

9 recurrent radial art.

10 radial N + d = deep branch

11 brachioradialis m

12 brachialis m

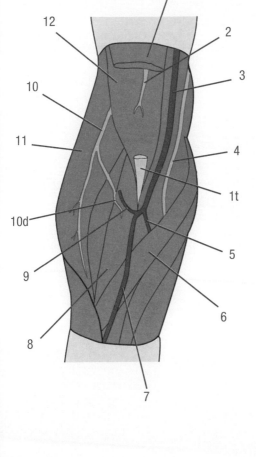

Blood supply of the Cubital fossa Superficial structures

Anterior – skin and superficial fascia removed

1   biceps (cut)   a = aponeurosis* m = muscle t = tendon

2   cephalic vein

3   brachial art.

4   median cubital vein

5   ulnar art.

6   pronator teres m

7   deep fascia

8   basilic vein*

9   medial epicondyle

10 brachioradialis m

* Biciptal aponeurosis is part of the deep fascia and pierced when sampling arterial blood from this area

* basilic and median cubital veins are common sites used for venupuncture. They along with the cephalic vein are part of the superficial venous network of the UL (similar to the saphenous vein and its brs in the LL). They are highly variable and travel in the superficial fat and fascia and are visible through the skin

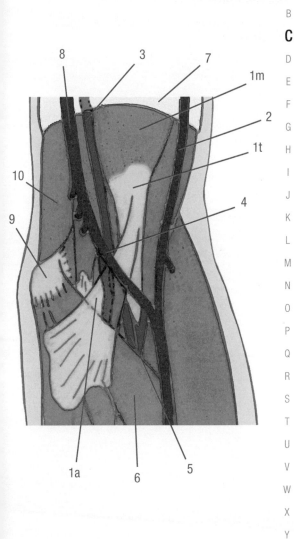

© A. L. Neill

Blood supply of the Diaphragm

Inferior view - looking up at the undersurface of the Diaphragm

The BS of the diaphragm unlike its NS comes from below and is from the 1st systemic paired branches of the abdominal aorta.

1 phrenic arteries R & L

2 opening in the central tendon for IVC

3 Sternum

4 oesophageal br of L phrenic art. to oesophagus efferent arterioles

5 anterior phrenic art. R & L

6 lateral phrenic art. R & L

7 medial and lateral arcuate ligaments

8 coeliac trunk

9 abdominal aorta

10 oesophageal opening in crura

11 central tendon

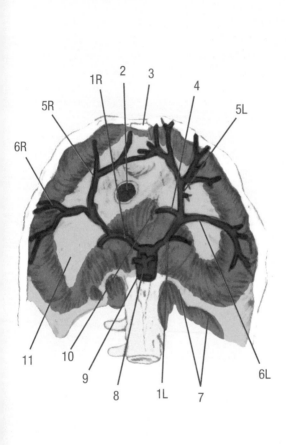

Blood supply of the Duodenum, Gall bladder, Pancreas & Spleen

Anterior view- stomach cut and removed – showing posterior structures behind the stomach most veins removed IVC remains

The stomach overlays the pancreas and duodenum, leaving a space behind, bordered by the omenta. The head of the pancreas lies in the curve of the duodenum. Branches of the coeliac trunk supply all these structures and richly aa. The pancreas is retroperitoneal.
The duodenum has its own mesentery.

1 spleen

2 L gastroepiploic art

3 splenic vessels

4 tail of the pancreas
    4a art. of the tail of the pancreas
    4d dorsal art. of the pancreas
    4g great pancreatic art.
    4h head of the pancreas
    4i inf. pancreatic art.

5 splenic art.

6 body of the pancreas

7 jejenum

8 middle colic art.

9 superior mesenteric vein

10 inf. pancreatoduodenal art

11 R gastro-epiploic art

12 duodenum

13 ant. sup. pancreatoduodenal art

14 supraduodenal art.

15 portal vein

16 common hepatic art.

17 coeliac trunk

18 gall bladder
    18c cystic art

19 branches of the proper hepatic art

20 gatric art L & R

21 inf. phrenic art

22 stomach – cut

A
B
C
D
E
F
G
H
I
J
K
L
M
N
O
P
Q
R
S
T
U
V
W
X
Y
Z

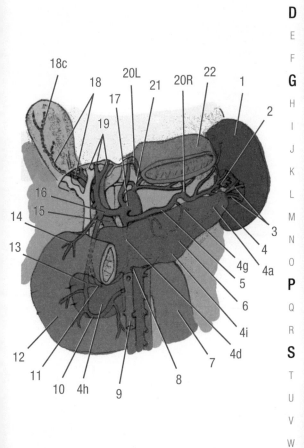

© A. L. Neill

Blood supply of the Ear

Arterial supply only

The BS of the ears: - the inner & middle ears are supplied from internal carotid brs.; the outer ear from brs. of the external carotid which via the supf. temporal art. has aas with the opposite side There are also aas b/n the int. & ext carotids.

1 supf. temporal art
2 ant. auricular art.
3 brs to the parotid gland
4 temporal art.
5 post. auricular art.
6 middle temporal art.
7 auricularis muscles
8 cochlea
9 labyrinthine art.
10 semicircular canals

© A. L. Neill

Blood supply of the Eye

Arterial supply of the Eyeball and internal structures

Upper- eyeball with CN II (optic N) removed
Lower - lens + anterior chamber of the eye

The BS of the eye has many components – eyeball, lens, retina and socket (which is part of the BS of the face).

1 ophthalmic art.

2 muscular brs. for extra-ocular muscles

3 lacrimal art.

4 central retinal art.
    i = inf br (this is deep to the sclera)
    r = retinal brs
    s = superior br

5 ciliary art. a = ant. br p = post. br

6 episcleral art.

7 major arterial circle - encircles the iris region
    coiled vessels

8 sclera

9 cornea

10 anterior chamber

11 dilator + constrictor muscles

12 iris

13 lens

14 pupil

Note: the cornea does not have a BS, but relies on diffusion from the anterior chamber

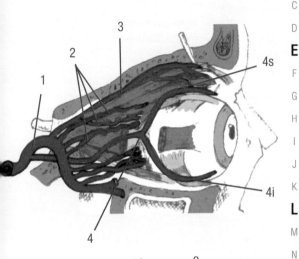

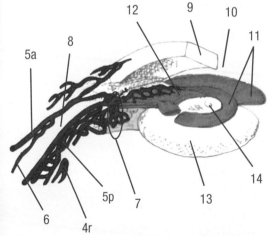

Blood supply of the Eye

Venours supply

Schema - lateral view
looking onto lateral wall of the R eye socket

Branches of the ophthalmic v drain the eye and its adnexae.

1 frontal sinus
2 supraorbital v
3 inferior ophthalmic v
4 facial v
5 Maxilla
6 maxillary sinus
7 pterygoid venous plexus
8 maxillary v
9 cavernous sinus
10 lacrimal v
11 long ciliary v
12 superior ophthalmic v
13 vorticose v (1 of 4 around the EB)

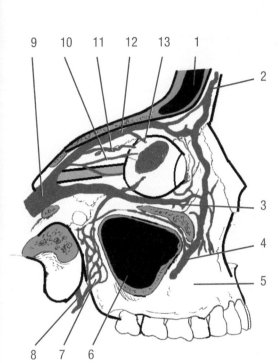

Blood supply of the Eyeball

Schema - surface views of the EB to show major arterial and venous systems

A lateral view of the EB

B anterior view of the EB

C anterior view of the cornea

The BS of the sclera must also supply the extraorbital muscles, conjunctiva & scleral fascia. The BVs are arranged in anastomotic circles similar to that in the brain. The veins also drain the aqueous humour of the anterior chamber, via a venous sinus as in the cerebrum.

1 minor arterial & venous circles

2 major arterial circle & sinus venous sclerae

3 radial v

4 ant. ciliarly a & v

5 long post. ciliary a + vorticose v

6 short post. ciliary a & v

7 episcleral venous plexus

8 intrascleral venous plexus

9 deep scleral plexus

10 venous collecting channel

11 aqueous v

12 ant. chamber

© A. L. Neill

Blood supply of the Foot

Arterial supply
Upper plantar
Lower dorsal

The BS of the foot relies on anastomotic arches similar to the hand - digits as with the hand are end arteries - hence subject to blockage anoxia and tissue death particularly so with diabetics.

1 first dorsal metatarsal art.

2 deep plantar arch

3 arcuate arteries

4 lateral tarsal art.

5 dorsalis pedis art.

6 plantar digital arteries

7 common plantar art.

8 plantar metatarsal art.

9 plantar arch

10 perforating arteries

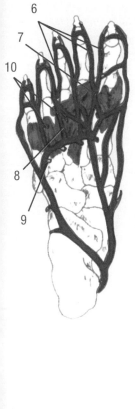

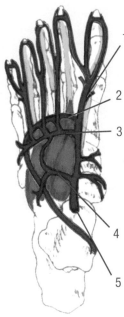

Blood supply of the Forearm

Arterial supply
Upper anterior/ventral surface (forearm) - palmer (hand)
Lower dorsal/posterior surface (forearm) - dorsal (hand)

The BS of the forearm comes from the terminal branches of the brachial art. the ulnar and radial arteries. The radial and ulnar arteries form the 2 palmar arches and the dorsal arch to supply the hand and fingers.

1   palmar arches d = deep / s = superficial

2   radial art. c = collateral

3   interosseus art. a = ant / c = common /
    p = post / r = recurrent

4   brachial art.

5   ulnar art. r = recurrent

6   dorsal carpal art. r = radial br / u = ulnar br

7   dorsal metacarpal art.

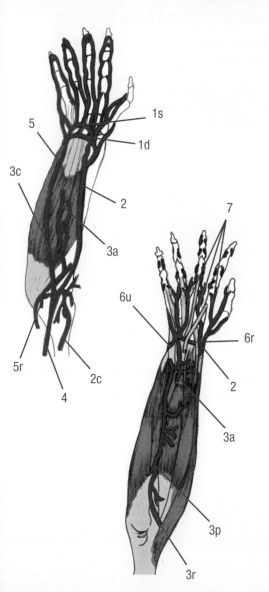

© A. L. Neill

Blood supply of the Hand and Wrist

Arterial supply
Palmar view - muscles, tendons & veins removed

The BS of the hand is made up of 2 anastomosing arches the deep and superficial palmar arches from which the digital vessels arise. The wrist is also supplied by the carpal arches which arise from the ulnar and radial arteries.

The fingers like toes do not have the rich arterial anastomoses around them seen in the elbow, hip, knee and shoulder joints. Their BS can be compromised by crushing, or blocking both sides of the digit.

1 radialis indicis = index br. of radial art
2 perforating brs of the deep palmar arch
3 princeps pollicis = principal thumb artery
4 deep palmar arch
5 superficial palmar branch of the radial art.
6 palmar carpal branches
   a = carpal arches
   r = of the radial art.
   u = of the ulnar art.
7 radial art
8 anterior interosseus art
9 ulnar art
10 deep palmar branch of the ulnar art
11 superficial palmar arch
12 common digital arteries
13 proper digital arteries

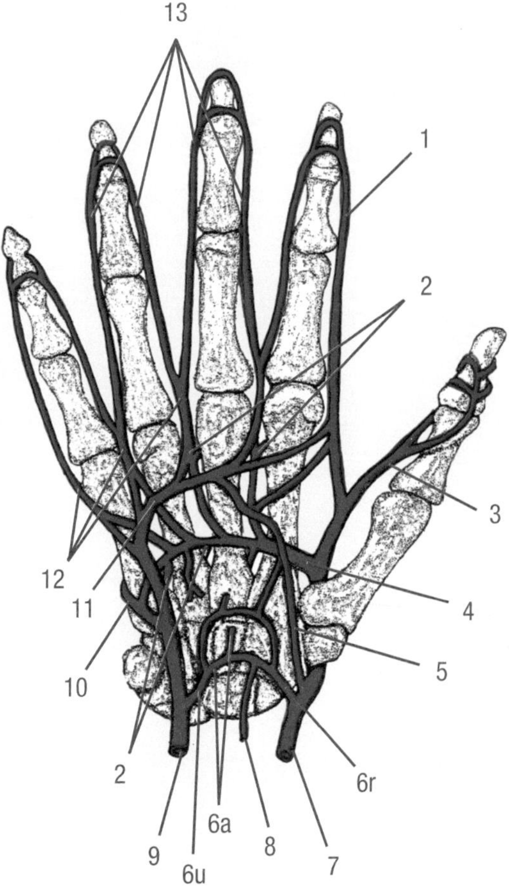
13
1
2
3
4
5
6r
7
8
6a
6u
9
2
10
11
12

Blood supply of the Head and Neck

Arterial supply - highly anastomotic

This is most important due to the poor definition of the fascial layers, the extensive mobility of the region, the concentration of Ns and special sensory structures.

The major supply of the extracranial BVs are from the external carotid. Supply also comes from the internal carotid and the vertebral arteries, and communication exists b/n all 3 sources.

Major Arteries of the Head and Neck
Anterior
Lateral

1 supraorbital

2 supratrochlear

3 frontal

4 parietal

5 zygomatico-orbital

6 infraorbital

7 transverse facial

8 ant. & post. auricular

9 external carotid from the common carotid

10 facial

11 mandibular → sublingual + submental branches

12 maxillary → superior + inferior alveolar branches

13 superfical temporal

14 middle temporal

15 labial vessels

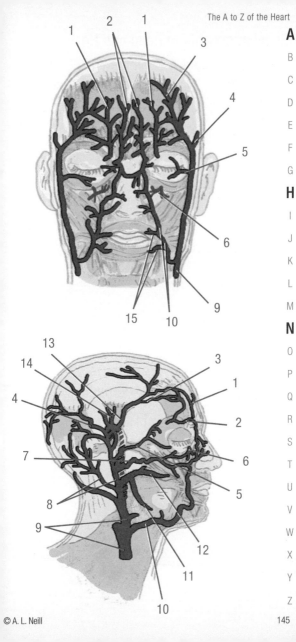

© A. L. Neill

Blood supply of the Head and Neck

Arterial supply - highly anastomotic

Major Arterial Anastomoses of the Head and Neck

1 AA b/n the supratrochlear / supraorbital / superficial temporal arteries from both the internal and external carotid arteries

2 AA b/n the anterior ethmoidal / maxillary branches and deep facial arteries in the nasal septum - (Little's area)

3 AA b/n the R & L and the upper & lower labial arteries

4 AA b/n the sublingual / submental /inferior alveolar arteries - all from the external carotid artery

5 AA b/n the superior and inferior thyroid arteries - from the external and common carotid arteries

6 AA b/n the ascending & deep cervical / vertebral arteries - from the aortic arch and common carotid artery

7 AA b/n the occipital and deep cervical arteries

8 AA b/n the posterior auricular / occipital / superficial temporal arteries - from the external carotid

9 AA b/n the superficial temporal arteries communicating b/n different sides of the scalp

10 AA b/n the deep temporal and the middle meningeal arteries -communicating b/n the extra-cranial and intra-cranial BSs

11 AA b/n the superficial and deep arteries of the face communicating b/n the fascial and muscle layers which are poorly defined in the face

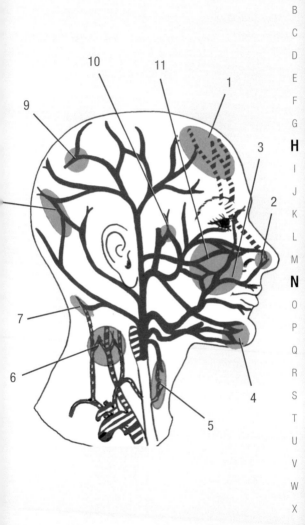

Blood supply of the Head and Neck

Venous drainage

Median plane - view looking into the R side of the head & neck
Skull, Maxilla and ½ the Mandible removed

1. sagittal sinus i = inferior / s = superior
2. lateral venous lacunae
3. emissary veins
4. arachnoid granulations
5. Parietal bone
6. straight sinus
7. petrosal sinus i = inferior / s = superior
8. transverse sinus
9. occipital sinus
10. occipital vein
11. retromandibular vein
12. post. ext. jugular vein
13. ext. jugular vein
14. internal jugular vein
15. R lymphatic thoracic duct
16. transverse cervical vein
17. suprascapular vein
18. R subclavian vein
19. R brachiocephalic vein
20. L brachiocephalic vein
21. inf. thyroid veins
22. thyroid
23. middle thyroid vein
24. superior thyroid vein
25. lingual vein
26. submental vein
27. facial vein
28. labial veins i = inferior / s = superior
29. pterygoid plexus
30. inf. alveolar vein
31. ext. nasal vein
32. inf. ophthalmic vein
33. angular vein
34. superior ophthalmic vein
35. supraorbital vein
36. supratrochlear vein
37. falx cerebri
38. cavernous sinus
39. great cerebral vein
40. maxillary vein
41. supf. temporal vein

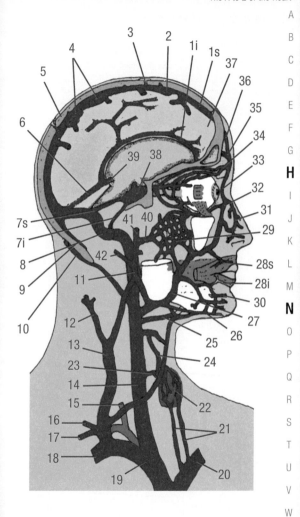

© A. L. Neill

Blood supply of the Hip

Arterial supply

Around the hip are extensive anastomoses to allow for the full range of movement of the limb w/o stopping the BS. Note several vessels change their names as they pass landmarks in the area i.e. the inguinal ligament

1 abdominal aorta

2 Iliac art c = common / e = external / i = internal

3 inguinal ligament (removed)

4 femoral art.

5 superficial epigastric

6 superficial circumflex iliac art.

7 tensor fascia lata m

8 circumflex arteries l = lateral / m = medial

9 perforating vessels

10 deep femoral art. = Profunda Femoris

11 external pudendal art.

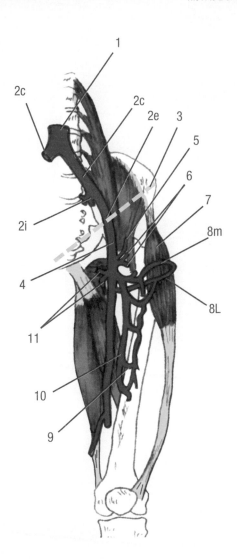

© A. L. Neill

Blood supply of the Jaws & Teeth

Schematic lateral view showing the arterial supply of the Mandible, Maxilla and the Teeth

Description: This diagram shows the intimate relationship b/n arteries of the teeth and other oral structures.

1 Middle meningeal a
  f = frontal br
  p = parietal br
  t = tympanic br
2 Sphenopalantine a
3 Infraorbital a
4 Post. sup. alveolar a
5 Descending palatine a
6 Buccal a
7 Pterygoid a
8 Masserteric a
9 Deep temporal a
10 Mylohyoid a
11 Tonsillar a
12 Dental a
13 Facial a
14 Mentala
15 Carotid a   c = common/ e = external/ i = internal
16 Ascending palatine a
17 Ascending pharyngeal a
18 Auricular a
19 Post. meningeal a
20 Maxillary a

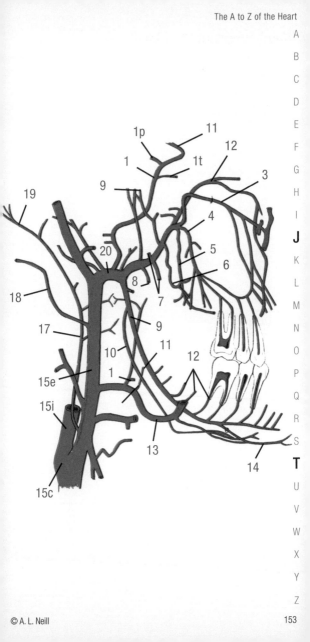

Blood supply of the Kidney

The renal BS is 20% of the CO. It has a HP BF and is a significant factor in determining the electrolyte and fluid level and balance in the body, and it filters the blood creating the urine in the process.

The individual unit of filtration is the nephron.

1 renal art.

2 segmental art.

3 interlobar art.

4 arcuate art.

5 interlobular art.

6 interlobular vein

7 arcuate vein

8 interlobar vein

9 segmental vein

10 renal vein

11 renal medulla

12 hilus

13 renal pyramid

14 renal cortex

15 renal capsule

16 renal pelvis

17 ureter

18 nephron

see also the nephron

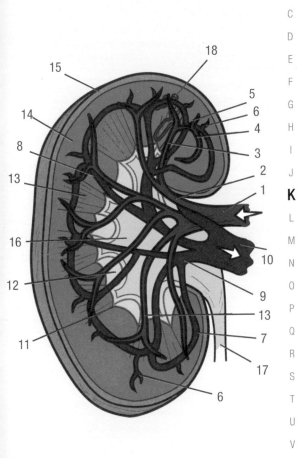

Blood supply of the Large Intestine (LI)

Arterial supply

LI spread out with retractors
mesentery and small intestine removed - note most of the LI is
retroperitineal ie attached to the back wall of the peritneum but the
transverse and sigmoid colons have separate mesenteries which support
their BS.

The BS of the LI is from the superior and inferior mesenteric arteries which anastomize with each other extensively. These are 2 of the 3 unpaired branches of the abdominal aorta - coeliac trunk opening only shown.

1 abdominal aorta

2 coeliac trunk

3 superior mesenteric art.

4 jeunal arteries

5 descending colon = L sided colon

5a L colic art.

6 ileal arteries

7 sigmoid colon

7a sigmoid arteries

8 rectum

8a superior rectal arteries

9 appendix

9a artery to the appendix (on a separate mesentery)

10 ileocolic art.

11 ascending colon = R sided colon

11a R colic art.

12 inferior pancreatoduodenal art.

13 middle colic art.

14 marginal art. = art. of Drummond

15 transverse colon

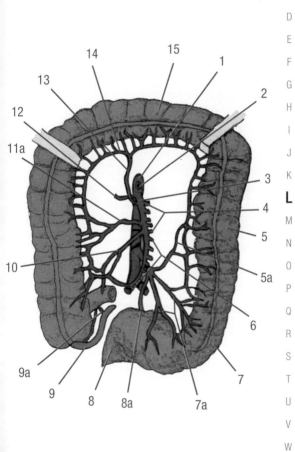

© A. L. Neill

Blood supply of the Larynx

Arterial supply

Lateral view with cartilage wall removed to show inside
Medial view - cartilage wall removed

The BS of the larynx, parathyroid and thyroid are related intimately. Hence voice changes may be a sign of pathologies in these areas.

1. carotid arteries c = common / e = external / i = internal
2. lingual arteries
3. hyoid arteries i = infrahyoid / s = suprahyoid art
4. laryngeal i = inferior / s = superior
5. thyroid art i = inferior / s = superior
6. cricothyroid m
7. thyrocervical trunk
8. subclavian art.
9. aorta
10. Hyoid bone
11. cricoid cartilage
12. epiglottis
13. thyroid
14. trachea

See also the thyroid

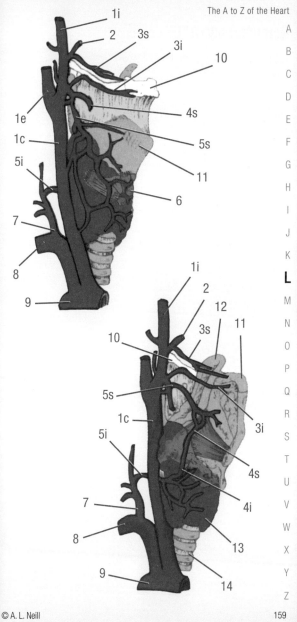

© A. L. Neill

Blood supply of the Liver

Upper – Anterior - schema of the BF
Lower – Inferior - view looking at the underside of the liver reflected upwards

The liver receives the GIT venous blood via the PORTAL vein. From there it drains to the IVC. The blood flows through the liver parenchyma via the sinusoids - open capillaries which allow for fluid, substance and cell movement into and out of the BVs. The arterial supply is via the hepatic artery which also drains to the IVC.

1   IVC

2   R & L hepatic veins

3   capillary network – sinusoids

4   cystic duct

5   hepatic artery

6   common bile duct

7   hepatic PORTAL vein

8   gall bladder

9   bile duct network

10 caudate lobe (BS – R hepatic art and vein)

11 R & L lobes of the liver

12 round ligament separating the R & L BS

13 quadrate lobe (BS – R hepatic art and vein)

14 Porta Hepatis = 5+6+7

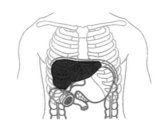

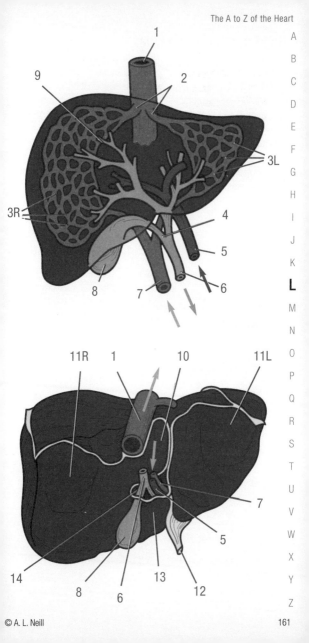

© A. L. Neill

Blood supply of the Liver Venous supply

anterior schematic overview

Definition: the liver is the largest organ in the body. It lies in the upper R quadrant. It is the major detoxifying organ – most of the absorbed material must first pass through this organ before entering the main BS. It also produces bile which assists greatly in fat digestion. In order to facilitate substances entering and leaving hepatocytes (liver cells), specially structured BF arranged in hexagonal lobules and veins – sinusoids – are unique features of this organ. This 4 lobed organ has great regenerative powers and generally weighs up to 2kg (4-5lb).

1   IVC

2   Hepatic vein L= left / R = right

3   Caudate hepatic vein (directly from IVC)

4   Superior hepatic vein L= left / R = right

5   Radial veins (radix veins) I = inferior / S = superior

6   anterior surface of the liver

7   Portal vein

8   distributing veins

9   Sinusoids

10 Central vein

11 Sublobular veins

12 posterior lateral hepatic vein

13 Middle hepatic vein – superficial

    A = arterial blood entering the liver – oxygenated

    B = bile leaving the liver to digest fat and lipids

    P = portal blood from the GIT - deoxygenated nutrient rich

    S = blood being detoxified through the sinusoids

    V = deoxygenated and detoxified blood returning to the body via the IVC

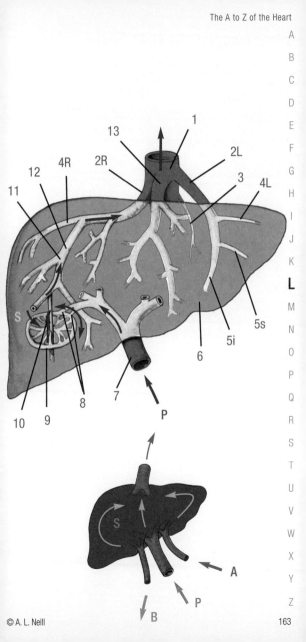

Blood supply of the Liver Sinusoids

Definition: the sinusoid is the specifically modified capillary of the liver. In order for substances to flow in and out with ease. The BM, a protein & fibrous network, and the endothelial cells lining the capillaries have large complete gaps and which allows protein to leave and blood including blood cells to move into the hepatocytes. Flow is slow and LP.

macroscopic schematic overview

1. Hepatic v
2. sinusoid p = peripheral, r = radial
3. interconnecting sinusoids / b/n hepatic lobules
4. venule sphincters i = inlet / o = outlet
5. distributing v
6. branch of Hepatic a
7. branch of Portal v
8. bile ductile
9. liver functioning unit – blood flows from here to the central vein (10)
10. central v
11. sublobular v = interlobular v

A = arterial blood entering the liver – oxygenated
B = bile leaving the liver to digest fat and lipids
P = portal blood from the GIT - deoxygenated nutrient rich
S = blood being detoxified through the sinusoids
V = deoxygenated and detoxified blood returning to the body via the IVC

microscopic schematic overview

1. BM
2. endothelial cell nucleus
3. cytoplasm of the endothelium
4. vacuole for transport of substances
5. RBC
6. cell to cell connection in endothelium
7. fenstration
8. gap in endothelium + BM

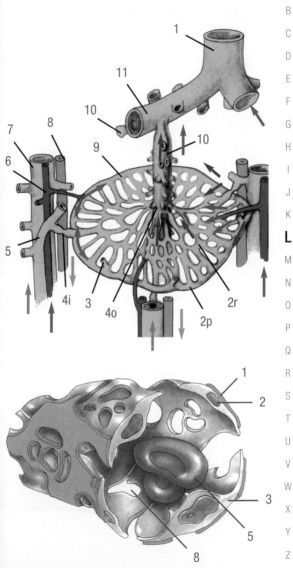

© A. L. Neill

Blood supply of the Lower Leg including major joints - Ankle & Knee

Arterial supply
Upper anterior
Lower posterior

Around the ankle and knee joints there are extensive anastomoses to allow for the full range of movement of the limb w/o stopping the BS. These arteries have an equivalent deep venous system.

1 popliteal art

2 tibial art.
   a = anterior / p = posterior

3 malleolar brs.
   L = lateral / m = medial
   note the anastomoses b/n these BVs

4 tarsal art.
   L = lateral / m = medial
   note the anastomoses b/n these BVs

5 dorsal artery of the foot

6 perforating br of the peroneal art.

7 anterior recurrent tibial art.

8 fibular circumflex art.

9 post. tibial recurrent art.

10 peroneal art.

11 communicating br of the peroneal art.

12 calcaneal art.

13 plantar art. L & m

14 nutrient art.

15 inferior geniculate art. L & m

16 superior geniculate art. L & m

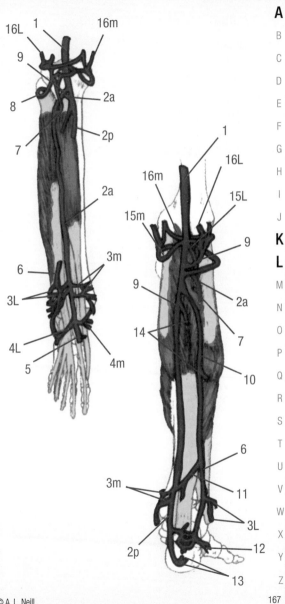

© A. L. Neill

Blood supply of the Lower Limb

Venous supply
Medial & Posterior – superficial veins

The superficial veins often present as varicose veins in the patient. They are hard to treat if ulceration has occurred, but may be removed without any clinical problems. Defective valves allow swelling and pooling of blood leading to thrombosis embolism pain & ulceration. Peripheral ischaemia, diabetes and other conditions also predispose to varicose veins. One common site is just below the emergence of the small saphenous vein from the deep fascia. Other sites are around the malleoli.

They are a separate system of veins which communicate with the deep veins via a series of perforating vessels. They do not have an arterial equivalent.

1 cribiform fascia
2 great saphenous vein
3 perforating veins
4 cut down site - medial malleoli brs
5 small saphenous vein
6 deep fascia
7 malleolus L = lateral / m = medial

* Yellow circles communication b/n deep and supf. systems through the deep fascia

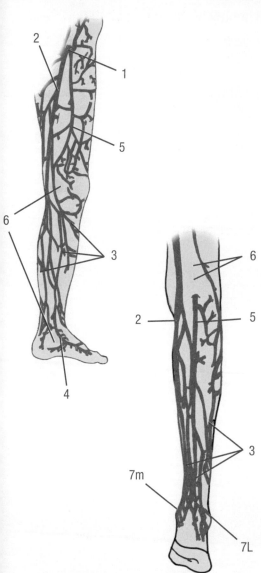

© A. L. Neill

Blood supply of the Lower Limb and Pelvis

Arterial supply
Anterior
Posterior - schema of arterial supply

This schema shows the relations b/n the hip and leg as well as the knee and lower leg with anastomotic networks around these main joints allowing for maximum movement with the least interference with BF. The leg has a deep and superficial venous supply - the deep supply following the arteries.

1. abdominal aorta
2. iliac / c = common / e = external / i = internal
3. superficial epigastric
4. superficial circumflex
5. circumflex brs of femoral artery / L = lateral / m = medial
6. perforating arteries
7. femoral / d = deep femoral
8. artery to the head of femur
9. external pudendal
10. obturator
11. tibial a = anterior / p = posterior
12. dorsalis pedis
13. tarsal arteries
14. gluteal art i = inferior / s = superior
15. cruciate anastomosis
16. geniculate anastomosis
17. popliteal
18. peroneal
19. plantar L = lateral / m = medial
20. metatarsal arteries

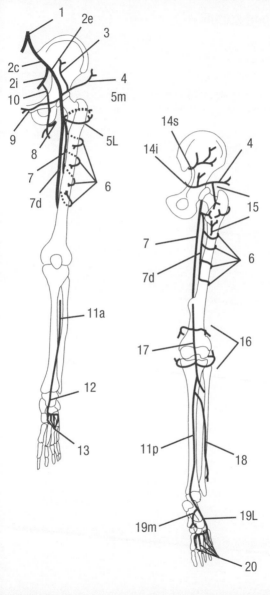

© A. L. Neill

Blood supply of the Lower Limb

Transverse
Lower leg = leg
Upper leg = thigh

This schema shows a transverse section through the upper and lower - leg, and the relationship with the compartments.

1 Tibia m = BM
2 great saphenous vein & N
3 e = EDL / f = FDL
4 nv of - Tibial N & post. tibial art & vein
5 subcut. fat
6 soleus m
7 peroneal art & vein
8 e = EHL / f = FHL
9 deep fascia extensions to demarcate the compartments of the LL
   i = interosseous membrane (leg only)
   ii - iii post. compartment leg - medial compartment thigh
   iii - iv lat. compartment leg - post compartment thigh
   iv – ii ant. compartment leg & thigh#
10 Peroneal muscles b = brevis / L = longus
11 Fibula
12 supf peroneal N
13 Peroneal N + ant. tibial art. & vein in nv bundle*
14 tibialis m a = ant. / p = post

15 profunda femoris art. + vein + Ns in nv bundle
16 sartorius m
17 femoral art. + vein + N to vastus medialis in nv bundle
18 obturator N
19 gracilis m
20 adductors / b = brevis / L = longus / m = magnus
21 semimembranous m
22 semitendinous m
23 biceps femoris m
24 sciatic N
25 gluteus maximus m
26 femur + BM (and Bone marrow)
27 vasti muscles i = intermedius / m = medialis / l = lateralis
28 rectus femoris m

*Note compression of the ant. compartment will result in compression of this nv

#note small lat compartment of thigh with tensor fascia lata not shown

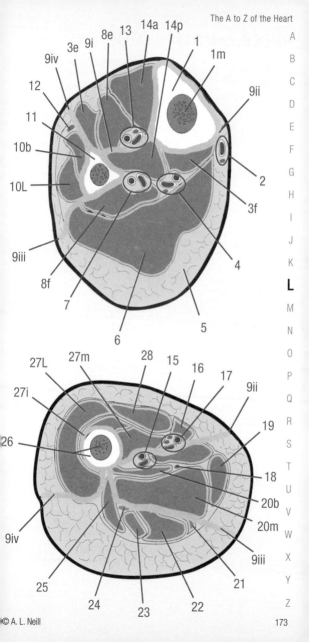

Blood Supply & Lymph Nodes of the Lungs

Arterial supply
Anterior view – Schema

The BS of the lung tissue arises from branches of the thoracic aorta and drains via the azygos system, as does the BS of the oesophagus in the upper ⅔. While cartilage itself does not have any BVs, the muscle and surrounding tissue obtain their nutrients supplied by these vessels.

LNs are found around all structures in these areas and freely drain from one group to another. The hilar and bronchogenic LNs are often implicated in lung cancer.

1 oesophagus

2 apex of the lung / L = Left / R = right

3 aorta / a = arch / t = thoracic

4 pleural br

5 2^0 bronchi / 1 for each lobe of the lung

6 root of the lung L = left / R = right - contains pulmonary arteries with deoxygenated B from the RV

7 oesophageal brs

8 bronchogenic LNs

9 hilar LNs

10 visceral pleura

11 aortic and para-aortic LNs

12 tracheal and para-tracheal LNs

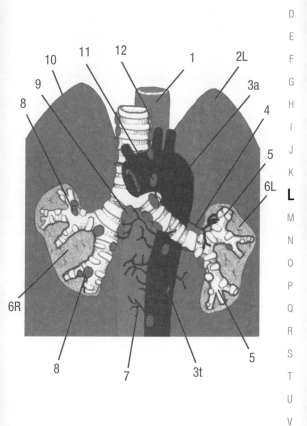

Blood supply of the Lymph node

Schema

LNs are bean-shaped organs in a fibrous capsule. Lymph enters the LN and is exposed to the lymphocytes in the outer cortex, progresses through to the medulla and then out via the efferent lymphatics of the hilum, after which it goes to further LNs in the group or to the CVS, via the thoracic ducts. Lymphocytes also leave via the post-capillary venules. The venules are lined with tall endothelial cells which have receptors to attract lymphocytes and facilitate their transport out of the LN. If any of the entering material is antigenic it will trigger the start of the immune reaction.

1 hilum vessels - artery, vein & efferent lymphatic

2 medullary sinuses & loose cords of lymphocytes

3 capsule and subcapsular sinus

4 lymphatic nodules (follicles) ± active (germinal) centres of lymphocyte proliferation

5 dense lymphocytic tissue of the cortex

6 deep cortex = paracortex

7 CT trabecula - with surrounding sinus

8 afferent lymphatics & valve

9 capillary network

10 post-capillary (high endothelial) venules

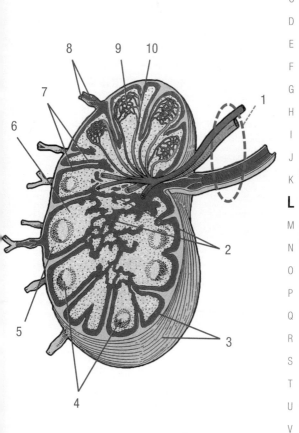

Blood Supply of the Mesentery

Schematic

Definition: the connective tissue fascial layer which surrounds the components of the GIT, and acts as the anchor to the posterior abdominal wall. It is derived from the peritoneum.

The stomach, transverse colon, appendix and sigmoid colon all have their own mesenteries, the rest of the GIT is fixed to the posterior wall of the abdomen. The mesentery allows for mobility of the gut and improves peristalsis – but it also allows for twisting and torsion of the gut, which may result in ischaemia and death of the twisted sections. Necrosis of the gut may result in perforation and release of the contents into the peritoneum – and peritonitis.

The greater omentum is 2 layers of the peritoneum fused together – and has a similar structure to mesenteric tissue.

1. SI
2. Vessels in the mesentery – note there are arteries veins and lymphatics
3. major art supplying the mesentery only arteries shown
4. connective tissue layer – generally a thin CT network with fat spread throughout but may act as a store for fat and be quite thick in obese patients

© A. L. Neill

Blood supply of the Nephron.
Renal unit of blood filtering

The nephron consisting of the glomerulus and is surrounding tubular network, filters the blood and forms the urine. It is the only BS to go from arterioles➡ capillaries➡ arterioles➡ capillaries➡ venules.

The urine is collected in the collecting ducts and accumulates in the renal pelvis.

1   interlobular artery and vein

2   afferent arteriole

3   glomerular capillaries

4   efferent arterioles

5   proximal convoluted tubules

6   peritubular capillary network

7   distal convoluted tubules

8   Loop of Henle – descending limb

9   base of the Loop of Henle

10 ascending limb of the Loop of Henle

11 collecting duct

12 Bowman's capsule = glomerular capsule

13 arcuate artery & vein

See also the Kidney

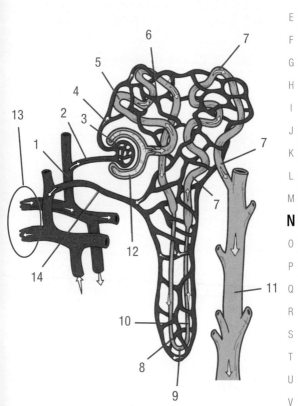

Blood supply of the Nose

Lateral view looking at the Conchae / Turbinates
Medial view looking at the Septum

The BS of the nose involves the joining of several BVs which anastomose in the septum and tip. This is a very well supplied area and prone to injury, and changes with hormones and other factors.

1 frontal sinus

2 lat. Nasal br of the facial art – to the ala of the nose

3 int. Nasal Br from V_2 (infraorbital N)

4 nasal conchae – turbinates
   i = inferior / m = middle / s = superior

5 nasal br of ant palantine N
   (from pterygopalantine ganglion)

6 pterygoid plate of the Sphenoid

7 sphenopalantine art (from maxillary)

8 post. ethmoidal art

9 ant ethmoidal art

10 ant ethmoidal N (V_1)

11 cut br of ant ethmoidal N – to tip of nose

12 subseptal art – from superior labial art (upper lip)

13 hard palate

14 sphenoidal sinus

15 nasalpalatine N (from pterygopalantine ganglion)

16 nasoseptal art (from 7)

17 ethmoid plate

18 Little's area site of anastomoses of several BVs - prone to haemorrhage

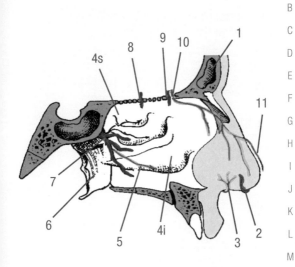

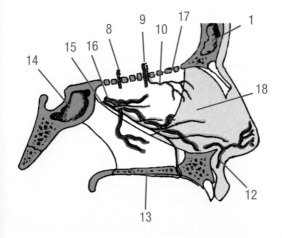

Blood supply of the Optic N & Retina

Transverse section through the Cerebrum LP
Longitudinal section through the Optic N (CNII) HP

1. central vessels of the retina a = artery v = vein
2. ophthalmic art.
3. internal carotid art.
4. cerebral arteries a = anterior / m = middle / p = posterior branches
5. lateral striate art.
6. optic radiation
7. visceral cortex
8. lateral geniculate body
9. optic N = CNII
10. basilar art.
11. anterior choroidal art.
12. communicating art. a = anterior / p = posterior
13. superior hypophysial art.
14. retina
15. choroid
16. sclera
17. short posterior ciliary arteries
18. DM
19. AM
20. PM
21. subarachnoid space
22. plial plexus
23. central collateral art.
24. circle of Zinn
25. lamina cribosa

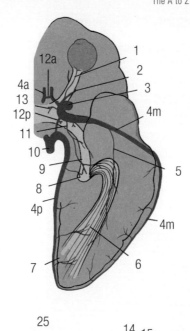

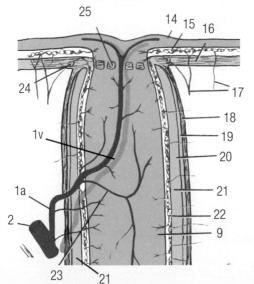

© A. L. Neill

Blood supply of the Ovary

Anterior – uterus straightened
Bladder & other organs removed - veins & ureter removed

The ovary sits in the peritoneal cavity and hence is susceptible to the consequences any events or infections of the peritoneum. Its rich BS anastomoses with that of the uterus, vagina and other structures of the pelvis. The ovarian artery is derived directly from the abdominal aorta, it travels down the abdomen as the foetus develops. In the male the BS moves further outside the the abdominal cavity altogether to follow the testis.

1   ovarian art.

2   suspensory lig. of the ovary

3   fimbria of fallopian tubes

4   ovary

5   uterine art.

6   vaginal art.

7   vagina

8   parietal peritoneum

9   fundus of the uterus

10 ovarian lig.

11 broad lig. (cut)

12 fallopian tube

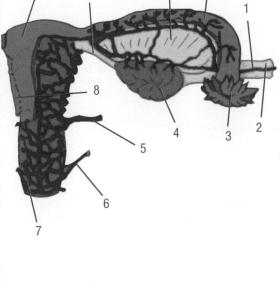

Blood supply of the Palm

Anterior view showing relationship b/n the arteries, Ns & tendons superficial

The BS of the palm is made up of anastomising arches which are arranged b/n layer of fascia and muscle hand is made up of 2 anastomosing arterial arches.

1 proper palmar digital art

2 princeps pollicus – principal thumb art.

3 superficial palmar brs of the radial art.

4 radial art
 d = deep br

5 ulnar art
 d = deep br

6 superficial palmar arch

7 common palmar digital art.

8 proper palmar digital art.

9 tendon of palmaris longus m

10 tendon of adductor longus m

11 ulnar N

12 median N

13 flexor retinaculum*

* Site of Carpal Tunnel Syndrome obstructing BV's and Ns

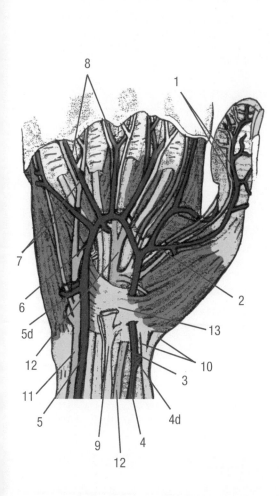

© A. L. Neill

Blood supply of the Pancreas and Spleen

posterior - *Arterial supply from the posterior aspect*

Description: the pancreas is intimately related to the spleen and duodenum and this is reflected in the BS.

1 Spleen
2 L gastroepiploic a
3 Short gastric a
4 Splenic a
5 Dorsopancreatic a
6 Coelic trunk
7 Common hepatic a
8 L & R Hepatic a
9 common bile duct a
10 Proper hepatic a
11 Supraduodenal a
12 Gastroduodenal a
13 R gastroepiploic a
14 Superior pancreato duodenal a
15 aas – branches
16 Duodenum – posterior surface
17 Anterior br (of the splenic a)
18 Post br
19 Inf. pancreato duodenal a
20 Superior mesenteric a
21 Inf. pancreatic a
22 Great pancreatic a
23 Pancreas – post aspect

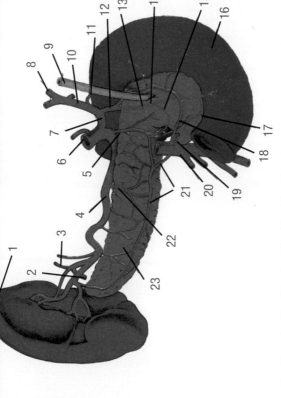

Blood supply of the Pancreas and Spleen

posterior - Venous supply from the posterior aspect

Description: the pancreas is intimately related to the spleen and duodenum and this is reflected in the BS. The Venous supply varies from the arterial as indicated but many aspects are mirrored.

1　Short gastric vessels

2　Splenic - in the groove on post surface of pancreas

3　Portal v

4　Common bile duct

5　Superior pancreato-duodenal veins

6　R gastroepiploic v

7　Duodenum post. surface

8　Inf. pancreato-duodenal v

9　Superior mesenteric v

10　Inferior mesenteric – note drains to the splenic v

11　Pancreatic brs

12　L gastroepiploic v

13　Multiple veins from the splenic hilum

A
B
C
D
E
F
G
H
I
J
K
L
M
N
O
P
Q
R
S
T
U
V
W
X
Y
Z

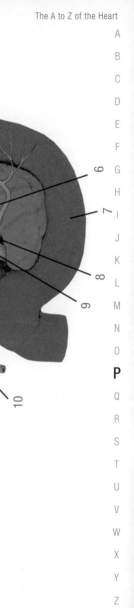

© A. L. Neill

Blood supply of the Pituitary Gland AKA Hypophysis

Arterial supply Sagittal schema

The Pituitary "gland" – is a dual organ, the anterior lobe (adenohypohysis) is an endocrine organ derived from the endoderm with sinusoidal vessels to carry the synthesized Hs to the body and the posterior lobe (neurohypophysis) an extension from the hypothalamus and so basically neural tissue. The BS is a series of capillary plexi which then reform portal vessels (arterioles) which break into sinusoids and glomeruli (knots) of caplliary plexi to absorb the Hs with maximum surface area and exposure and then distribute these substances. Two axes of communication are thus facilitated - an efficient access from the hypothalamus to the anterior lobe of the pituitary, and from the pituitary to the body.

1   internal carotid a

2   superior hypophyseal a

3   hypophyseal portal v

4   hypophyseal v

5   secondary plexus - sinusoidal capillaries in the ant lobe

6   inferior hypophyseal a & v

7   middle lobe = pars intermedia

8   infundibulum

9   primary plexus - sinusoidal capillaries of the hypothalamus

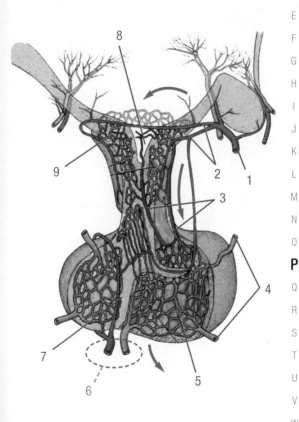

Blood supply of the Popliteal fossa = posterior knee & posterior ankle

Arterial supply

Around the knee are extensive anastomoses to allow for the full range of movement of the limb w/o stopping the BS. The large popliteal artery surrounded by muscles of the posterior leg is the site of the popliteal pulse.

1 Femur

2 descending br of lateral circumflex femoral art

3 popliteal art

4 superior geniculate art L = lateral br / m = medial br

5 fibular collateral ligament

6 Inferior geniculate art L = lateral br / m = medial br

7 descending geniculate art

8 femoral art

9 tibial collateral ligament

10 ant. tibial recurrent art

11 fibular circumflex art

12 tibial art. a = anterior / p = posterior brs

13 interosseus membrane

14 fibular art = peroneal art

15 malleolar art L = lateral br from peroneal art /
   m = medial br from post. tibial art

16 calcaneal br

17 dosalis pedis

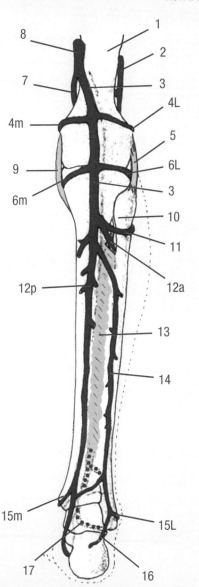

8
1
7
2
4m
3
9
4L
6m
5
6L
3
12p
10
11
12a
13
14
15m
15L
17
16

© A. L. Neill

Blood supply of the Retina

View of the normal features of the back of the EB - retina

The integrity of the back of the eye is viewed directly using the ophthalmoscope with or without a dilated pupil.

1 OD containing the central retinal BVs – central retinal artey & vein

2 inf nasal retinal v

3 inf temporal retinal a

4 macula

5 fovea

6 superior temporal retinal a

7 superior nasal retinal v

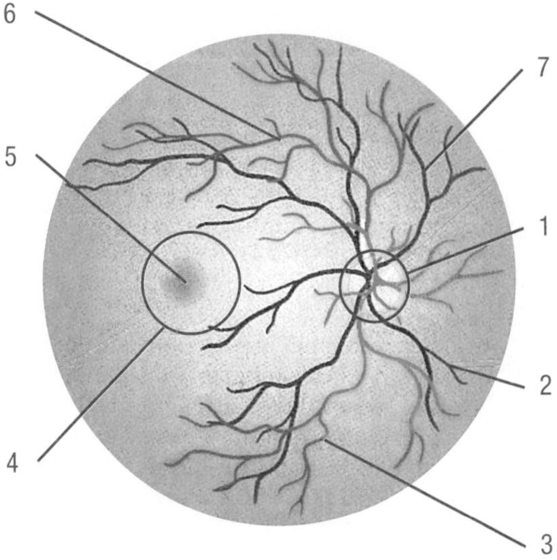
6
7
5
1
2
4
3

Blood supply of the Rib – thoracic segment

Microscopic MP

The BS of the ribs are segmental like many thoracic structures

1   thoracic aorta

2   azygos vein

3   SC

4   post. IC artery & vein

5   post. perforating IC art. & post. br of
    the dorsal N

6   lat. br of the IC art. & N

7   innermost IC muscles (intercostal intimi)

8   costal groove on the rib

9   collateral brs of the IC art. & vein

10 anterior IC nv

11 Xiphoid process

12 anterior perforating art & vein

13 ant. cutaneous br. of the IC N

14 internal thoracic art & vein = ant. mammary art & vein

15 Sternum

16 Manubrium

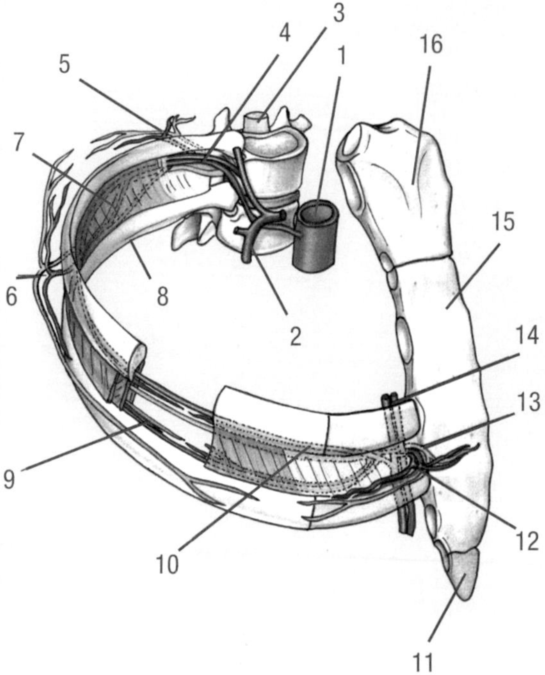

A B C D E F G H I J K L M N O P Q R S T U V W X Y Z

Blood supply of the Scapula

Arterial supply
Posterior view

1 suprascapular art.

2 Clavicle

3 Acromion

4 axillary art.

5 circumflex scapular art.

6 brachial art.

7 teres m

8 anastomoses with intercostal art.

9 rhomboid m

10 levator scapulae m

11 transverse cervical art.

12 subclavian art.

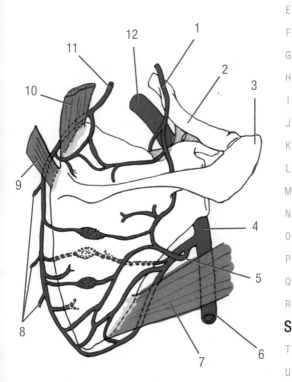

Blood supply of the Shoulder

Arterial supply
Posterior - superficial

1 suprascapular art & N

2 acromion

3 deltoid m

4 axillary N

5 posterior circumflex humeral art

6 Humerus

7 brachial art d = deep branch (profunda brachii)

8 radial N

9 triceps m

10 teres muscles major & minor

11 circumflex br of the subscapular art.

12 infraspinatus m

13 Spine of Scapula

14 supraspinatus m

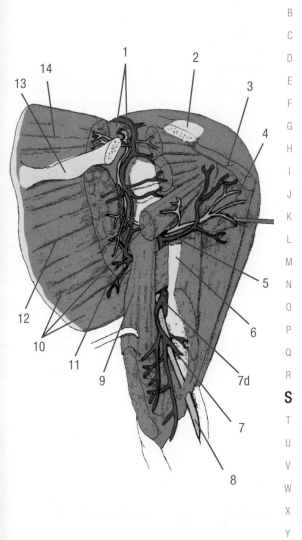

Blood supply of the Spinal Cord

Schema of the SC anterior surface and cross section

C = cerebral region
T = thoracic region
L = lumbar region

1   basilar art.

2   vertebral art.

3   radial artery of C5

4   radial artery of C7

5   anterior spinal art.

6   lateral thoracic arteries

7   artery of the lumbar enlargement
    expanded on the one side at the level of T10 – L2

Spinal Cord

Schema of the SC – deep and superficial arterial networks

Note there are minimal anastomoses b/n these 2 different circulations

This circulation as with the brain has end arteries and distally the tissue may be compromised.

A   deep arterial network – neural tissue supplied by ant. spinal artery

B   superficial arterial network

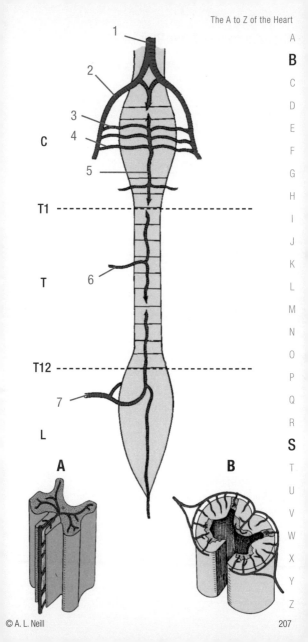

1

2

3

4

C

5

T1

T

6

T12

7

L

A

B

© A. L. Neill

Blood supply of the Stomach

Anterior – in situ – liver and pancreas removed

The stomach is supplied by branches of the coeliac trunk and has extensive anastomoses on both the lesser and greater curves with the joining of the L & R gastric vessels and the L & R gastroepiploic vessels, and drains via the portal system to the liver.

1 oesophagus coming through the diaphragm
   oesophageal br. of the L gastric art.

2 fundus of the stomach

3 L gastro-epiploic art

4 short gastric vessels

5 spleen

6 splenic art. (runs across the top of the pancreas)

7 greater omentum

8 gastro-epiploic R & L aa

9 gastroduodenal art

10 duodenum + stomach pyloris

11 gall bladder

12 cystic artery

13 portal vein + R hepatic duct

14 common hepatic art.

15 R gastric art.

16 coeliac trunk

17 space in the central tendon of the diaphragm
   for the IVC

18 L gastric art.

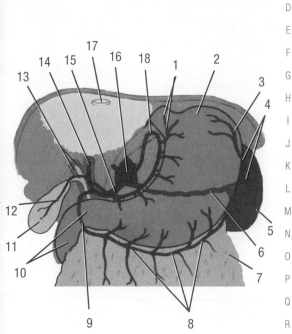

Blood supply of the Temporomandibular joint (TMJ)

The TMJ is very sensitive to irritation, art, veins and Ns are in juxtaposition near an unstable joint which moves through a large ROM

1 deep temporal

2 lateral pterygoid m

3 maxillary

4 buccal N

5 buccinator m

6 Mandible

7 masseter m

8 facial

9 ext jugular

10 sternocleidomastoid m

11 retromandibular v

12 inferior alveolar a & N

13 facial N

14 sphenomandibular ligament

15 superficial temporal a & v

16 auriculotemporal N

© A. L. Neill

Blood supply of the Testis

Outline of the BS of the spermatic cord, testis and testicular layers with the parenchyma removed

The testis is one of the male organs of reproduction - forming and releasing the sperm in the seminiferous tubules. The scrotum houses the testes and is surrounded by muscles and CT layers to protect the organ as it lies outside the body, in order to allow the sperm to mature which they cannot do at body temperature.

1 Testicular a & v

2 Ductus deferens a &v

3 Cremateric a & v

4 Seminiferous tubule arterioles & capillaries

5 pampiniform plexus

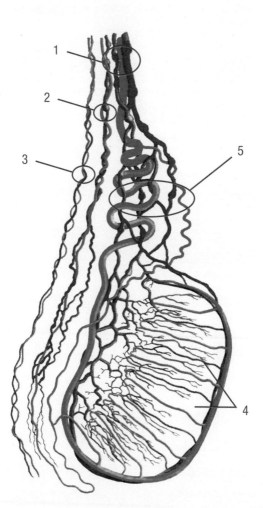

© A. L. Neill

Blood supply of the Thymus

A *Anterior view of the thymus in the mediastinum with the thyroid gland removed*

B *Schema of the microcirculation demonstrating*

The thymus is part of the immune system and supplies T lymphocytes. The circulation resembles that of the LNs. The blood flows around the capsule and courses through the cortex filtering through the Blood-Thymic-Barrier. It occupies the anterior mediastinum lying anterior to the pericardium. It is b/n 20-30gms in the child but with age degenerates and may not be discernible in the adult.

1 L jugular v

2 L subclavian v

3 L internal thoracic a & v (AKA mammary)

4 L phrenic N + pericardiophrenic a

5 anterior pericardium

6 thymus anterior surface

7 thymic a

8 superior vena cava

9 R brachiocephalic v (AKA innominate)

10 trachea

11 thymic arteriole (from thymic a)

12 thymic capsule

13 Thymus-Blood-Barrier

14 post-capillary v

15 corticomedullary junction (arcuate vessels)

16 medulla

17 thymic venule

18 efferent lymphatic

19 medullary capillaries

A

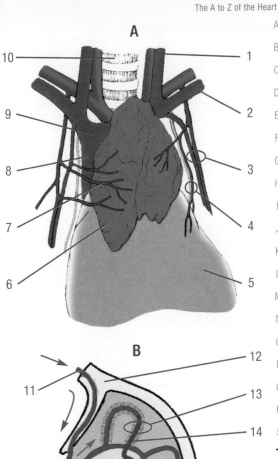

B

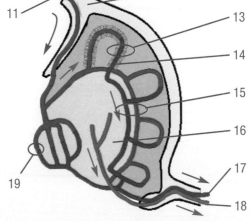

Blood supply of the Thyroid

Anterior view of the thyroid gland

The thyroid is an endocrine gland hence the BS is copious and the capillaries open to secretions. It is usually supplied via 3 paired branches from the carotid artery, draining into the internal jugular vein.

1 common carotid a

2 internal jugular v

3 superior thyroid a & v

4 thyroid gland - pyramidal lobe

5 thyroid isthmus

6 thyroid ima a

7 brachiocephalic v

8 brachiocephalic v

9 trachea

10 inf thyroid a

11 middle thyroid v

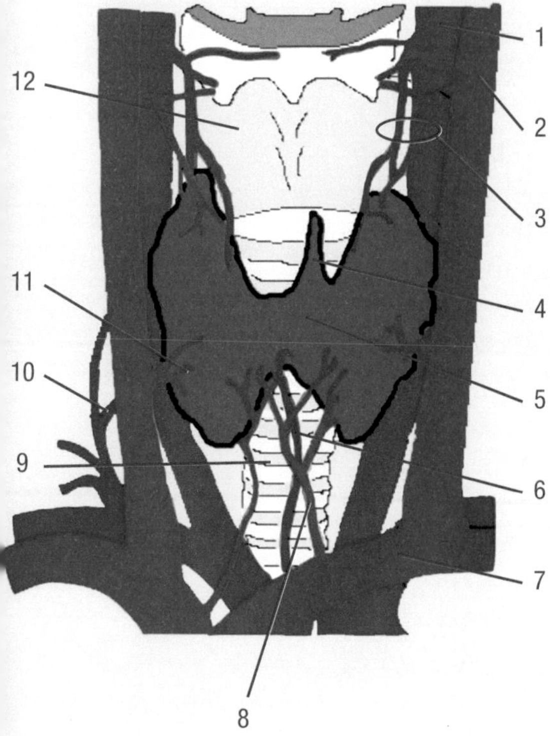
1
2
3
4
5
6
7
8
9
10
11
12

Blood supply of the Thyroid & Parathyroid glands

Arterial supply
Anterior
Posterior

1. Thyrohyoid muscles
2. superior thyroid art.
3. lateral lobe of the thyroid
4. inferior thyroid art.
5. thyrocervical trunk
6. subclavian art.
7. common carotid art
8. aortic arch
9. L bronchus
10. Thyroidea ima art.
11. isthmus of the thyroid
12. pyramidal lobe of the thyroid
13. parathyroid gland i = inferior / s = superior
14. trachea
15. nasal cavity
16. uvula
17. oral cavity with tongue

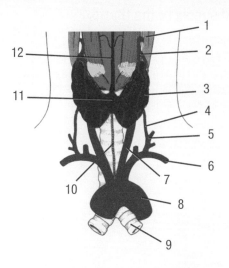

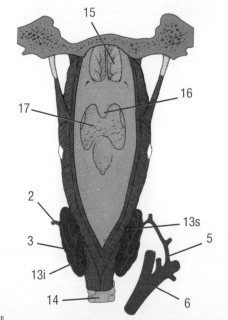

© A. L. Neill

Blood supply of the Uterus

Anterior

The BS of the uterus and vagina are intimately related and there is an extensive anastomosis b/n them. The uterine artery and vein are also closely related to the ureter and this clinically significant in surgical procedures such as hysterectomy.

1 fundus

2 fallopian tube = ovarian tube = uterine tube

3 ovarian ligament

4 broad ligament

5 uterine art. & vein R & L

6 ureter

7 vaginal art. and vein

8 rugae

9 vagina

10 cervix

11 uterine cavity – lined by endometrium

12 myometrium – muscle of the uterus

13 ovarian art. & vein R & L

14 tubal cavity

15 body of the uterus

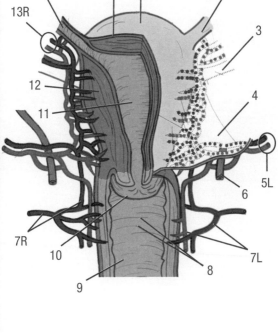

© A. L. Neill

Blood supply of the Uterus

Relations with the ureter
Anterior - in situ

uterine vein and ovarian vessels removed
Parietal peritoneal covering cut away to show structures underneath

The BS of the uterus and ureter are closely related – note the coiled uterine artery

1 ureter R & L

2 rectum / sigmoid colon

3 fundus of the uterus

4 fallopian tube = uterine tube

5 ovary + ovarian ligament (note ovary is in the peritoneal cavity)

6 parietal peritoneum

7 external iliac art. + vein

8 round ligament (of the uterus)

9 utero-vesical pouch

10 recto-uterine pouch = Pouch of Douglas

11 bladder

12 internal iliac art.

13 fat in the pelvic cavity

14 uterine art.

15 IVC

16 abdominal aorta

A
B
C
D
E
F
G
H
I
J
K
L
M
N
O
P
Q
R
S
T
U
V
W
X
Y
Z

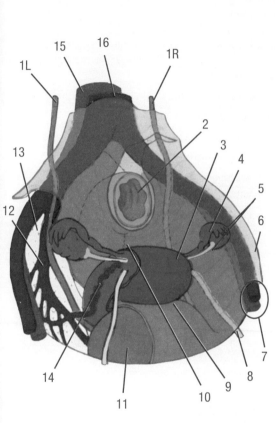

© A. L. Neill

223

Blood supply of the Uterus

Schema

The BS of the uterus comes from branches on the internal iliac and is intimately related to that of the adjacent structures, such as the vaginal BVs from the hypogastric. The intimate relationship b/n the uterine and the ureter is important to note - particularly in procedures such as an hysterectomy.

1   uterus - fundus

2   ovarian tube

3   ampulla

4   ovarian a - br from the aorta

5   ovary

6   ureter

7   internal iliac a

       p = internal pudendal

       m = middle rectal

       u = uterine

       v = vaginal

8   perineal a

9   vestibule

10 cervix

A
B
C
D
E
F
G
H
I
J
K
L
M
N
O
P
Q
R
S
T
U
V
W
X
Y
Z

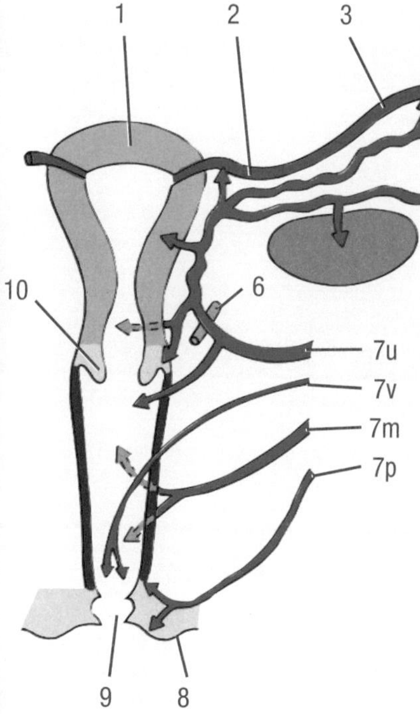

Blood Supply of the Vertebrae

Superior view - arteries
veins
Lateral view - veins

The vertebral column and vertebrae are supplied via segmental spinal branches from the aorta and iliacs and branches from the azygos network of vessels. The BS is richly anastomotic. The body of the vertebrae has red bone marrow and continues to form blood cells into adult life.

1 SP

2 TP

3 vertebral foramen

4 VB

5 pedicle

6A spinal artery

6V intravertebral vein

7 intercostal artery / vein

8A segmental artery

8V intervertebral vein

9 basivertebral vein

10 venous plexus of vertebral body

11 anterior venous plexus

12 posterior venous plexus

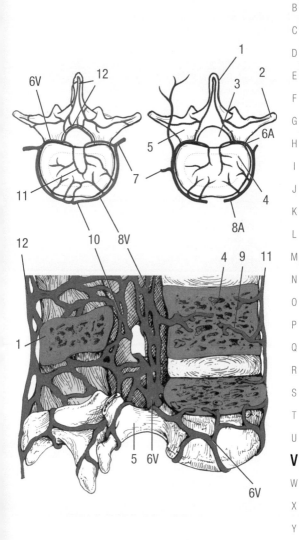

The Aorta – development

4 weeks
5 weeks
The arterial system has become closed and circulates throughout the embryo and placenta.

There are 3 paired aortic arches which develop into the single aortic arch.

The 3 unpaired branches of the abdominal aorta have formed and begun to supply the growing GIT system.

1. embryo
2. dorsal aortae
3. aortic arch
4. umbilical arteries
5. unpaired branch of the dorsal aorta
6. dorsal aorta –abdominal
7. truncus arteriosus
8. coeliac trunk
9. dorsal mesentery
10. superior mesenteric art
11. inferior mesenteric art
12. internal iliac art – to supply the pelvis
13. external iliac art – to supply the developing LL
14. small intestines
15. liver
16. diaphragm
17. thoracic cavity
18. oesophagus

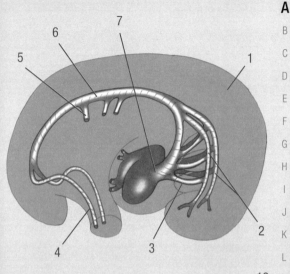

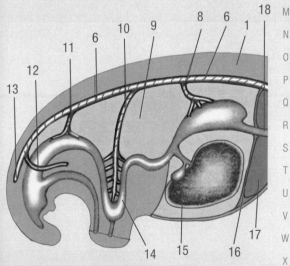

© A. L. Neill

Aorta – abdominal

Major branches
Anterior view - schema.

The abdominal aorta is bound superiorly by the diaphragm and terminates as the common iliac arteries at the level of L5.

The branches of the abdominal aorta can be grouped as follows:

1-3 are Parietal paired branches ↑P

1　Inferior Phrenic art.
2　Lumbar art. from L1-4
3　Common iliac art.

4　is an unpaired parietal branch ↑P

4　Median sacral art

5-7 are unpaired Visceral branches – ↓P (portal system)

5　Coeliac trunk
6　Superior mesenteric art
7　Inferior mesenteric trunk

8-9 are Visceral paired branches ↑P

8　Renal arteries
8a　Adrenal arteries
9　Gonadal art. (ovarian in females / testicular in males)

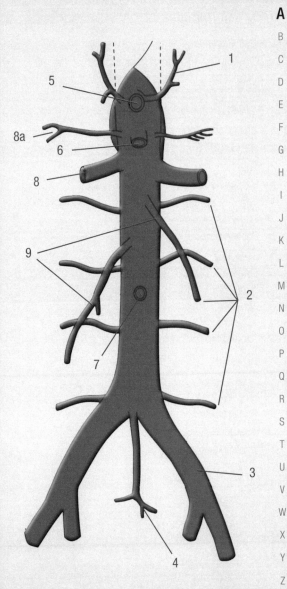

© A. L. Neill

Aorta – abdominal

Circulation schema

The abdominal aorta has 2 main types of branches - the parietal - supplying structures of the abdominal wall and the visceral - supplying contents in the abdomen -

1-4 are Parietal branches - paired

1   Inferior Phrenic art.

2   Lumbar art. from L1-4

3   Common iliac art. (terminal brs)

4   Median sacral art

5-7 are unpaired Visceral branches – and part of the ↓P portal system

5   Coeliac trunk

51 L gastric

52 Splenic – 521 – Pancreatic / 522 – L gastroepiploic / 523 – short gastric

53 Common Hepatic – 531 – Hepatic art. proper / 532 – R gastric / 533 – gastroduodenal

6   Superior mesenteric art

61 inf. pancreatoduodenal

62 jejunal

63 ileocolic

64 R colic

65 middle colic

7   Inferior mesenteric trunk

71 L colic

72 sigmoid

73 superior rectal

8-9 are paired Systemic branches - part of the ↓P Systemic circulation

8   Renal arteries - 81 - adrenal

9   Gonadal art. (ovarian in females / testicular in males)

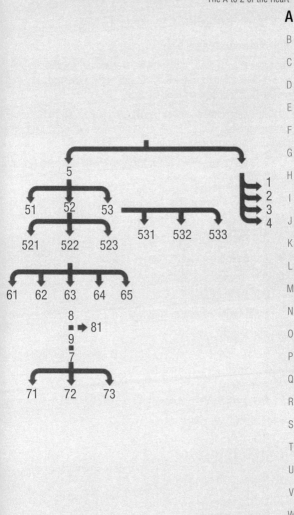

Aorta – Thoracic

Anterior view – heart, lungs, lymphatic and veins removed

The thoracic aorta lies in the posterior mediastinum which can be further divided into the ascending aorta, the arch of the aorta and the descending aorta (above the diaphragm)

It is highly segmental and branches supply the ribs & intercostal spaces, the oesophagus, trachea and bronchi as well as the lung pleural tissues and the pericardium.

Note the vasa vasorum (BVs of the BVs) also arise here and supply the aorta itself

1   oesophagus

2   L common carotid and subclavian arteries

3   arch of the aorta

4   Carina (point if bifurcation of the trachea)

5   brs arising from the aorta o = oesophageal /
    p = pericardial

6   diaphragm – central ligament

7   opening for the IVC

8   IC art. – part of the IC nv which is from above down
    V = vein
    A = artery
    N = nerve

9   R main bronchi (note more vertical than the L)

10 BVs supplying the R bronchus

11 trachea

12 R brachiocephalic artery

13 innermost IC muscles

14 internal IC muscles

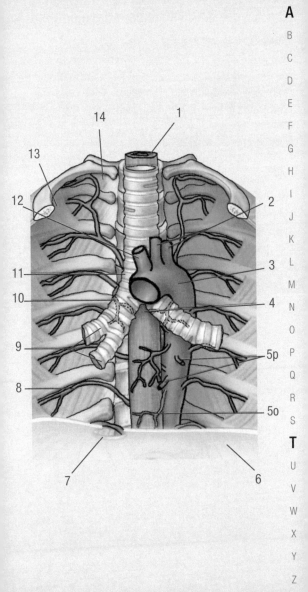

The Azygos & Caval veins – development

6 weeks
New born

The venous system like the arterial is originally symmetrical but then develops on the opposite side to the arterial system – the R. The supplementary venous supply - the azygos system remains and forms an alternative to drainage via the IVC and the SVC.

1 Anterior cardinal veins persist as... the jugular veins

2 Common cardinal vein moves to the R and persists as... SVC

3 subcardinal veins persist with some deterioration on the L as... the Azygos system with the azygos (a) and hemiazygos (h) veins

4 posterior cardinal veins

5 R posterior cardinal vein persists as... the IVC

6 Iliac anastomoses persist as ...
Internal (i) and external (e) iliacs and pelvic plexi

7 adrenal vein

8 renal vein

9 gonadal vein

10 gonad – female = ovary / male = testis

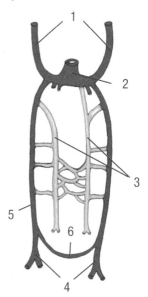

© A. L. Neill

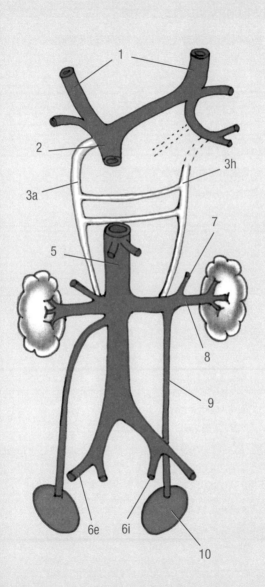

Cavernous venous sinus

Superior view - looking at the base of the skull

Coronal view - looking through the sinus - at the level of the red line

The cranial venous drainage is via a number of slow flowing venous lakes - or sinuses. These thin-walled amuscular channels receive CSF from arachnoid granulations. The cavernous sinus positioned superior to the sphenoid sinus is intimately related to the arterial & nerve supply of the eye, as well as part of its venous drainage.

1   intercavernous sinus

2   cavernous sinus

3   basilar venous plexus

4   marginal sinus

5   confluence of the cranial venous sinuses

6   sigmoid sinus

7   inferior & superior petrosal sinuses

8   sphenoparietal sinus

9   ophthalmic veins

10 pituitary gld

11 internal carotid a

12 CN II - optic N

13 CN III - oculomotor N

14 CN IV -trochlear N

15 CN V divisions 1 & 2 = ophthalmic N (i) & maxillary N (ii)

16 CN VI - abducens N

17 Temporal lobe

18 sphenoid air sinus

19 nasal cavity

20 Sphenoid b

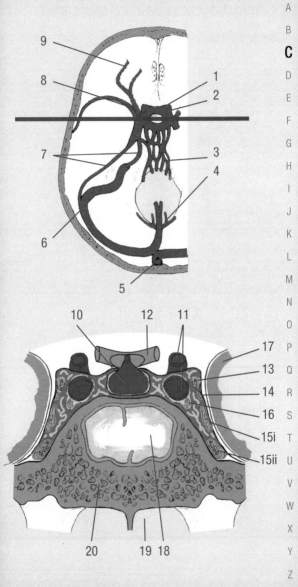

Circle of Willis = Cerebral arterial circle

Microscopic MP

Arterial vessels to supply the cerebrum arise from the inferior surface of the brain via the internal carotid arteries which enter the cranium via the carotid canal and the anterior surface of the SC via the Basilar artery from the fusion of the 2 Vertebral arteries. These 3 BVs form an anastomotic arterial ring - the circle of Willis - from which branches arise to supply the cerebrum. Because of its structure, supply can be continued despite the blockage of any 1 or 2 of the individual contributors, provided it is not acute. However distal to the ring this is not the case.

1 Anterior cerebral
2 Anterior communicating
3 Ophthalmic
4 Internal carotid
5 Medial striate
6 Middle cerebral
7 Lateral striate
8 Anterior choroid
9 Posterior communicating
10 Posterior cerebral
11 Superior cerebellar
12 Posterior choroid
13 Basilar

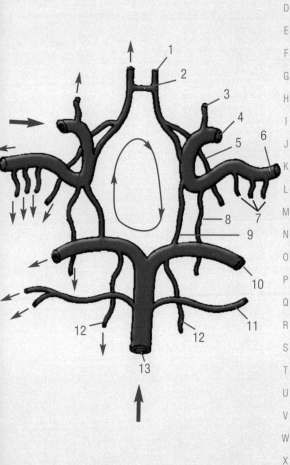

© A. L. Neill

Coeliac Trunk = Celiac Trunk

The first unbranched artery arising from the abdominal aorta, part of the GIT BS. It supplies the lower end of the oesophagus stomach and duodenum. The branches of the superior mesenteric and the coeliac art have a number of variations – the commonest are demonstrated here.

1. Fundus of the stomach
2. Diaphragm
3. Spleen
4. Gastroepiploic art. L = left , R = right
5. Aorta
6. Gastroduodenal a
7. Common hepatic a
8. Gastric art L = left, R = right
9. Coeliac trunk
10. IVC
11. R crus of the diaphragm
12. Oesophagus
13. Physiological sphincter of the diaphragm
14. Splenic a
15. Renal a – note this is not part of the GIT BS
16. Superior mesenteric a
17. Hepatic art. L = left, R = right branches

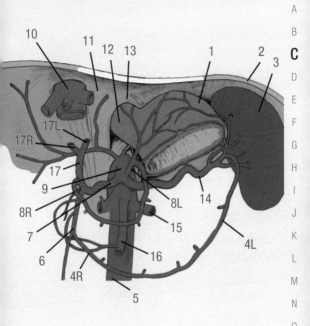

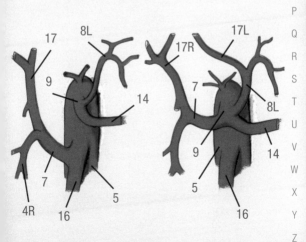

© A. L. Neill

IVC

Major branches
Anterior view- schema

The Vena Cava is a large vein split in 2 the SVC above the heart draining into the RA and the IVC below draining into the RA.

This BV may be endangered with herniated discs.

The branches of the IVC show common variations from R to L

1-2 are hepatic vessels

1   middle hepatic vein

2L left hepatic vein – drains the L lobe of the liver

2R right hepatic vein – large vein -drains the large R lobe of the liver

3   inferior phrenic veins R & L drain the diaphragm equally

4-6 drain the adrenal renal and gonads

4L L adrenal vein drains to the L renal vein

4R R adrenal vein drains to the IVC

5L single vein - 2 br.

5R double vessel – no br.

6L L gonadal* drains to the renal vein

6R R gonadal drains to the IVC

7   form the IVC

7L 3 br. int. & ext. iliacs and median sacral unpaired vein (10)

7R 2 br. int. & ext iliacs

8   external iliac veins

9   internal iliac veins

In females the ovarian and in males the testicular veins

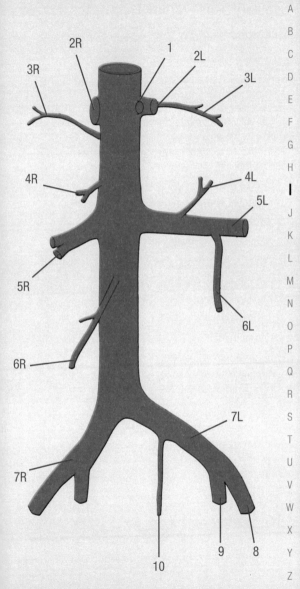

© A. L. Neill

Capillary beds – arteriole

Microscopic MP
Closed capillary bed
Open capillary bed

In most tissues there are many capillary beds with as few as 5% open at any one time open - e.g. the skin. Changes in the BF through these areas are stimulated by: hormones, local metabolites, oxygen levels, the ANS and other factors, but this in all cases is mediated by the arteriole (1) system which by a series of sphincters (3) directs the BF either into the beds (8) or to bypass (5) them and go directly to the venous system (6).

1 arteriole
   taking B away from the heart ↓

2 metarteriole

3 precapillary sphincter – c = closed / o = open

4 capillary – reduced size when the bed is isolated

5 throughfare / capillary bed bypass

6 venule
   bringing B to the heart ↑

7 smooth muscle cells

   - dense on arterioles /
   - sparse on venuoles /
   - absent on capillaries

8 capillary bed

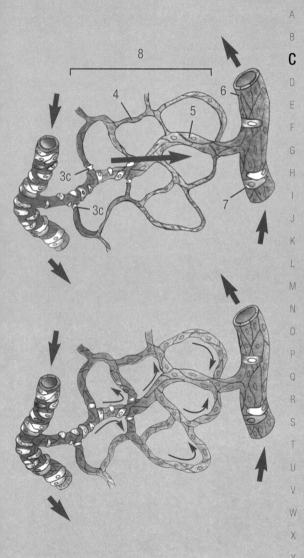

Capillary beds
Arteriole → Lymphatic + Venule

Microscopic MP

Capillary bed showing the role of the lymphatic drainage. Fluid and protein remains in the tissue and is not returned to the veins for draining. This fluid moves into the lymphatics to be filtered and returns via the thoracic ducts.

1. arteriole
2. tissue - cells
3. capillary bed -
4. lymphatic capillary
5. venule
6. collagen fibre - attached to cm - pulls the lymphatic open when the T swells

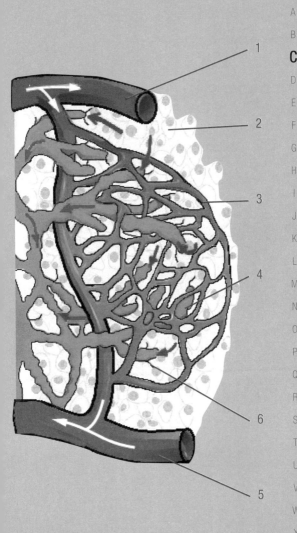

Cardiac cycle

Definition: All the events associated with a single heart beat

The heart consists of 4 chambers - 2 atria and 2 ventricles, which fill and empty together in the cardiac cycle.

1   RELAXATION PERIOD – both the A & V are relaxed and the Atria receive blood from either the body or the lungs

2   VENTRICULAR FILLING – with the changes in P the AV valves open and the RV & LV fill to 75%

3   ATRIAL SYSTOLE – to complete the Ven filling, the Artia contract and complete the last 25% of ventricular filling.

4   VENTRICULAR SYSTOLE – the Ven contract opening the semilunar aortic and pulmonary valves and shutting the AV valves LUBB (1ST HEART SOUND) and emptying the ventricles.

The Ventricles RELAX -

1   shutting the semilunar valves DUBB (2ND HEART SOUND) and beginning the cycle again.

Hence the HS are LUBB DUBB / LUBB DUBB etc.

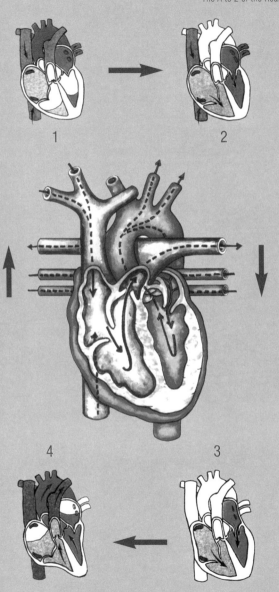

Circulation of the Heart
coronary arteries

Anterior view of the coronary arteries and the cardiac veins
The pulmonary trunk has been removed and the heart rendered transparent to show the BV rings forming around the heart

20% of the CO is used to supply the heart itself - 2 main branches arise from the ascending aorta,(L&R) which further branch to form 2 arterial rings

1 forming b/n the atria & the ventricles and 1 dividing the LV & RV

From these rings come the "terminal" branches which supply the myocardium. Hence blockages may occur in the rings and still not compromise the BS to the heart (unless acute) but more distal blocks will result in myocardial death.

1 aortic arch

2 pulmonary trunk (removed)

3 R auricle

4 RA (post.)

5 RV (ant + post)

6 descending aorta / thoracic aorta

7 LV

8 IVC

9 LA

10 SVC

11 ascending aorta

12 L coronary artery

13 R coronary art. / small cardiac vein

14 L circumflex art. (br of the L coronary art.)

15 ant. interventricular art (br of L coronary art.) / great cardiac vein

16 post. interventricular art (br of R coronary art.) / middle cardiac vein

17 marginal coronary art. / anterior cardiac vein = small cardiac veins

18 Coronary sinus

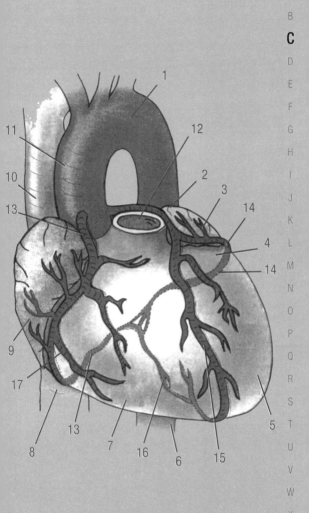

Circulation of the Heart
cardiac veins

Anterior view of the coronary arteries and the cardiac veins
The pulmonary trunk has been removed and the heart rendered transparent to show the BV rings forming around the heart

The cardiac veins mainly follow the coronary arteries and drain into the coronary sinus – on the post. surface of the heart b/n the A and ven. It is an amuscular sac, which needs the heart contraction to empty its contents directly into the RA.

1 aortic arch
2 pulmonary trunk (removed)
3 R auricle
4 RA (post.)
5 RV (ant + post)
6 descending aorta / thoracic aorta
7 LV
8 IVC
9 LA
10 SVC
11 ascending aorta
12 L coronary art.
13 R coronary art.
/ small cardiac vein
14 L circumflex art. (br of the L coronary art.)
15 ant. interventricular art (br of L coronary art.)
/ great cardiac vein
16 post. interventricular art (br of R coronary art.)
/ middle cardiac vein
17 marginal coronary art.
/ anterior cardiac vein = small cardiac veins
18 Coronary sinus

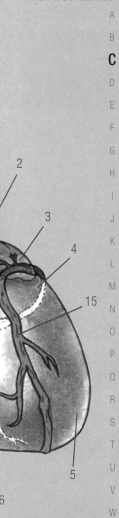

Foetal circulation
Major bypasses

Anterior view- schema

In the foetal circulation the O_2 and nutrients come from the placenta – hence the pulmonary circulation is bypassed in the foetus via the ductus arteriosus and the common atrial cavity which diverts B away from the lungs back to the aorta. The ductus venosus diverts B away from the liver and gut tissues to the IVC directly.

1   SVC

2a aortic arch

2d descending aorta

3   ductus arteriosus

4   pulmonary trunk

4a pulmonary arteries

4v pulmonary veins

5   lungs – collapsed in the foetus

6a umbilical arteries

6v umbilical veins

7   ductus venosus

8   IVC

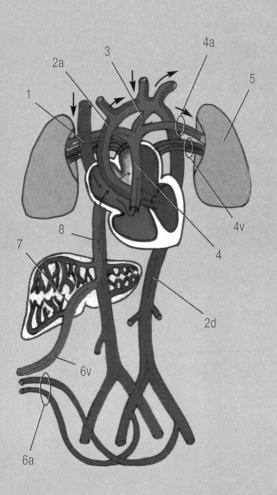

© A. L. Neill

Foetal circulation – detail
Liver

Development of liver bypass
Upper view 6 weeks – sinusoids
Lower view 8 weeks – ductus venosus

In the foetal circulation the liver develops a low pressure pooling sinusoidal system, however with the rapid growth of the foetus and the food supply from the placenta this is temporarily bypassed - by a large duct - ductus venosus which collapses again after birth

1 sinus venosus

2 stomach

3 L & R vitelline veins - forming hepatocardiac channels

5 sinusoids

6 umbilical vein

7 portal vein (from fusion of 3)

8 vitelline veins draining to the liver
   (later to form mesentery vessels)

9 duodenum

10 cardinal vein

11 Hepatic portion of IVC (from fusion of 3)

12 ductus venosus (bypass of sinusoids)

13 pancreas

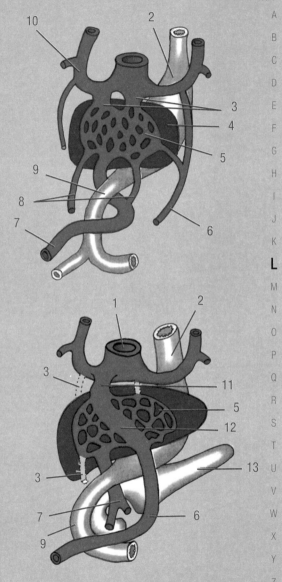

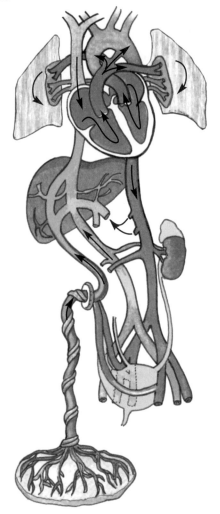

circulation of the foetus

Main oxygen and nutrient supply via the umbilicus, Pressure even
throughout, essentially 1 atrium, B mixes throughout via arterial and
venous shunts

© A. L. Neill

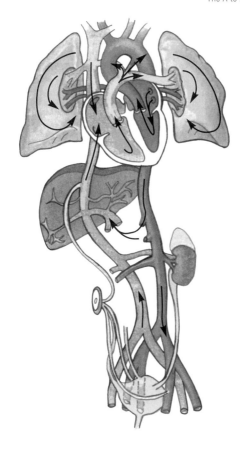

circulation of the newborn

Oxygen now from the lungs and nutrients from the GIT – umbilicus shuts down, lungs expand, shunts close, circulations separate - ↓ pressure on R side and ↑ pressure on the L

Pulmonary Circulation

Schema

The cycle of the R- sided or pulmonary circulation is needed to oxygenate the blood for the rest of the body.

1 RV empties ...

2 ...filling the Pulmonary trunk

3 R & L pulmonary arteries carry the B to...

4 ...the R & L lungs

5 B is exposed to O_2 in the capillary beds/alveoli of the lungs ... OXYGENATED

6 ...R & L pulmonary veins return the B to the

7 L atria..

8 ...and then the Lventricle
   where B is then taken to the rest of the body

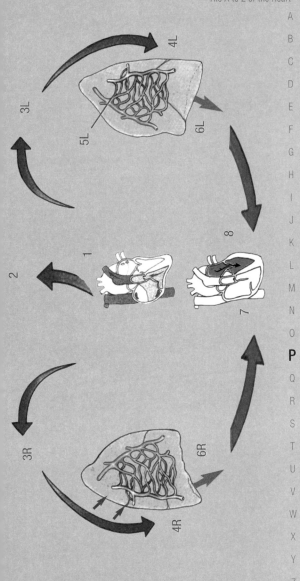

4L

3L

5L

6L

8

2

1

7

3R

6R

4R

© A. L. Neill

Heart Circulation
Left side - Systemic

Schema

The circulation has 3 main components – art., venous and lymphatic.

Arteries are defined as vessels taking B away from the heart

Veins as vessels bringing B to the heart & lymphatics as returning extra vascular fluid to the heart

Simultaneously all 3 components are moving fluid or B around the body in their defined pathway.

	arteries	veins	lymphatics
no of vessels	+	++	+++
valves	–	+	++++
pressure	++++	++	+/–
wall thickness	+++++	+++	+

1 RA
2 RV
3 R & L pulmonary arteries
4 Pulmonary capillary beds
4A Lymphatic capillary beds
5 Pulmonary veins
5A Pulmonary lymphatic vessels
5B Pulmonary LNs
5C Lymphatic valves
6A LA
7 LV
8 Aorta

9 Systemic arteries
10 Systemic capillary beds
10A Lymphatic capillary beds
11 Systemic veins
11A Systemic lymphatic vessels
11B Systemic LNs
11C Systemic lymphatic valves
12 IVC
12A systemic lymphatic drainage ducts.

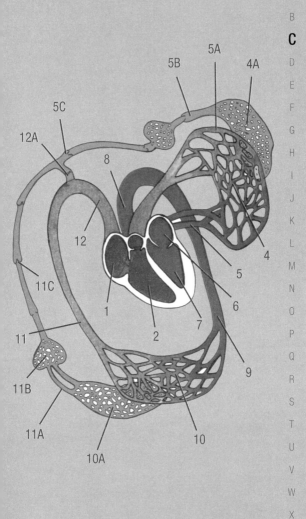

Lymphatic drainage

Anterior view – posterior thoracic wall
Aorta and azygos system removed

The posterior mediastinum forms part of the posterior thoracic wall. The lymphatics drain each ICS and form large ducts to empty at the intersection of the jugular and subclavian veins on the L & R.

1   duct emptying into L subclavian & jugular veins

2   L subclavian vein

3   rib

4   Thoracic duct = L lymphatic duct

5   LNs

6   lymphatic vessels

7   lumbar lymphatic trunks L & R

8   intestinal lymphatic trunk

9   cisterna chyli

10 R thoracic duct = R lymphatic duct

11 SVC

12 duct emptying into R subclavian & jugular veins

13 R jugular vein

14 oesophagus

15 L common carotid art and L jugular vein

© A. L. Neill

Lymphatics
relationships with the major BVs

Anterior view –

Lymphatics flank most of the major BVs draining to interconnecting groups in the axilla, inguinal region and the trachea.

1   cervical LNs and vessels

2   thoracic duct L & R

3   subclavian vein L & R

4   tracheal and bronchogenic LNs – often involved in "lung" cancer

5   axillary LNs (major area of drainage of the ant chest wall and breast)

6   lumbar LNs and vessels

7   pelvic LNS

8   inguinal LNs and vessels

9   cisterna chyli

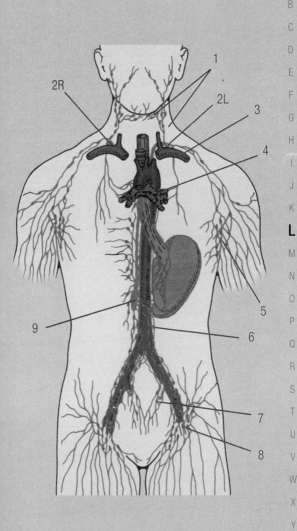

Lymphatics – overview
Drainage

Anterior view – schema

The R thoracic duct drains approximately a quarter of the body including half the head and neck region while the L drains the rest. The spleen, tonsils, Peyer's patches of the SI and BM all have a relationship with the lymphatic system.

1 submandibular LN
2 cervical LNs and vessels
3 spleen
4 Peyer's patches in the SI
5 inguinal LNs and vessels
6 BM red at the ends of long bones
7 cisterna chyli
8 epitrochlear LN
9 mammary LNs drain to the ...
10 axillary LNs
11 palatine tonsil
12 thymus

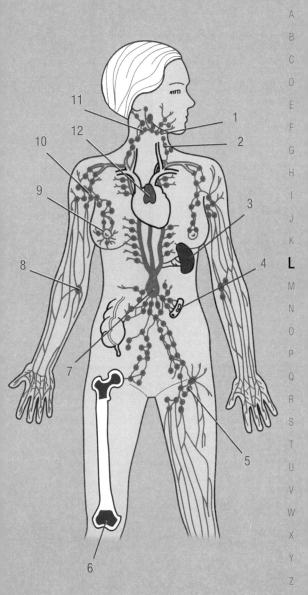

© A. L. Neill

Portal – Systemic anastomoses

Schema

Where the portal and systemic circulations meet there may be a pressure differential particularly in disease states and varicosities or distensions of the portal veins may occur, which if they rupture can lead to serious haemorrhages.

1. azygos vein
2. oesophageal vein draining to azygos vein
3. oesophageal vein draining to L gastric vein
4. stomach + oesophagus
5. portal / systemic aa = 3 + 2
   site of oesophageal varicosities
6. splenic vein
7. inf. mesenteric vein
8. superior mesenteric vein
9. venous drainage of LI and lower GIT
10. superior rectal vein -draining to inf mesenteric
11. inferior rectal – draining to int. iliac veins
12. portal / systemic aa = 10 + 11
    site of haemorrhoids
13. anus
14. epigastric veins superior + inferior
15. paraumbilical veins
16. portal / systemic aa = 14 + 15
    site of "caput medusa"- ring vessels on the abdominal wall
17. liver
18. IVC

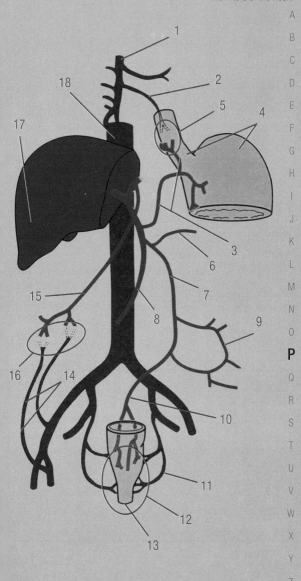

Vena Cavae = IVC + SVC
Collateral vessels - bypass circulations

Schema showing blood draining into the heart (removed) from the SVC and IVC

Primarily the systemic venous return is via the VCs – however 3 other collaterals exist mainly the Azygos/hemiazygos circulation which also feeds from the vertebral venous plexus. Others include the supf abdominal and thoracic vessels draining to the veins of the UL and portal system via the liver.

1   jugular veins from the H&N draining to the SVC

2   vertebral venous plexus

3   segmental veins

4   azygos system + hemiazygos BVs

5   veins from the LL

6   supf epigastric

7   portal circulation draining to IVC

8   internal + lateral thoracic veins

9   subclavian + axillary veins

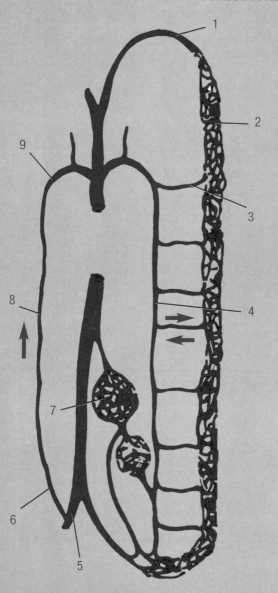

© A. L. Neill

Auscultation –
listening to the heart & CVS

Anterior chest wall = Praecordium

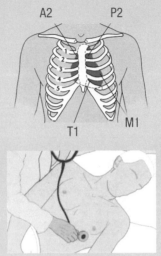

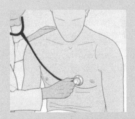

Listening to the apex beat and mitral valve

Listening to the heart base and aortic valve

Listen for the sounds of the closure of the 4 Heart valves associated with cardiac cycle events. The sounds radiate to areas on the ant chest wall - heart sounds (HS) 1 and 2

A2 - aortic area / M1 - mitral area / P2 - pulmonary area / T1 - tricuspid area

© A. L. Neill

Heart Sounds and Murmurs
Definition sounds associated with the cardiac cycle

They are also associated with jugular venous pressure (JVP) changes and cardiac cycle events.

a = atrial contration
c = tricuspid valve closure
v = atrial filling
y = rapid ventricular filling

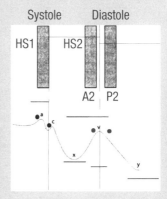

There are 2 classic Heart Sounds (HS) associated with the noise of the valves closing – commonly described as LUB, DUB – HS1 = the closure of the L&R AV valves (M1, T1) , best heard at the apex; HS2 = the Aortic (A2)and Pulmonary (P2) semilunar valves closing, best heard at the base.

Additional sounds occurring b/n HS1 & HS2 = SYSTOLIC MURMURs – the commonest are due to aortic stenosis & mitral regurgitation

Additional sounds occurring b/n HS2 & HS1 = DIASTOLIC MURMURs – the commonest are due to aortic regurgitation & mitral stenosis

HS3 = mid-diastolic murmur –
    normal in high BF situations eg pregnancy
    Pathological in L ven failure and valve regurgitation
    syndromes

HS34 = late diastolic murmur – always pathological

METALLIC SOUNDS of prosthetic valves

OS = opening snap – in mitral stenosis

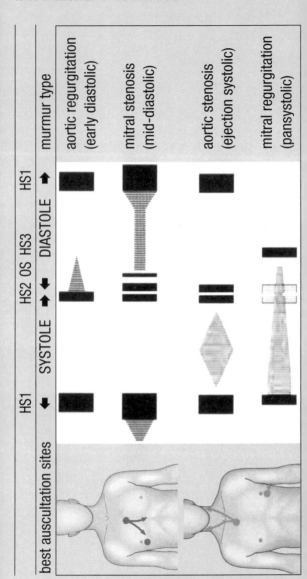

© A. L. Neill

Clinical Examination of the Heart and CVS

Inspection

When first looking at the patient observe the following:

Whole body observations

breathlessness at rest (CHF), pallor (anaemia) or cyanosis (cardiac failure),

hands - shake hands - temperature- hot / cold clammy (peripheral cyanosis) - pale, purple fingers

xanothamata - fatty plaques on the skin and around the tendons - ($\uparrow$ cholesterol $\pm$ $\uparrow$ fats and lipids)

legs swollen redness on the back of the legs - (DVT = deep vein thrombosis)

ankles - swollen ankles - (peripheral oedema)

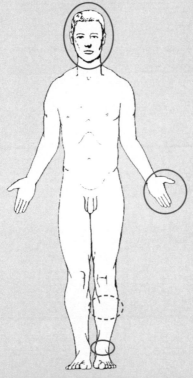

Chest anterior = Praecordium

Surface landmarks of the chest include

1 MCL – site of the apex beat
2 pacemaker site
3 apex beat observe heaves of enlarged heart lateral to this
4 site of liver ptsosis and congestion due CCF
5 parasternal heaves – RV hypertrophy
6 median sterniotomy scar – open heart surgery
7 manubriosternal joint and sternal angle
8 jugular notch

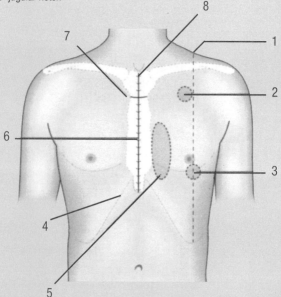

© A. L. Neill

Face

Eyes - anaemia - look under the eyelid for pallor, arcus corneae - (white ring around edge of the cornea indicates lipid deposits) xanthelasma - yellow plaques around the eyelids

Cheeks - malar flush - red butterfy pattern on the cheeks

Lips and tongue - central cynaosis - purple grey lips and bluey purple tongue

Palate - highly arched in Marfans - associated with congenital heart disorders

Teeth - decay a possible site for infective endocarditis

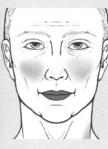 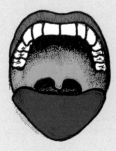

Nails

Nail changes may indicate CVS and other pathology

NAD		Clubbing	koiloncyia = spoon nails	splinter hae-morrhages	pitting
heart disease		infective endocarditis congenital heart cyanosis	iron deficiency anaemia	infective endocarditis	
other disease assoc		carcinoma of the bronchus lung abscess liver cirrhosis congenital	congenital	hard labour injury to hand -	psoriasis

Also look for tobacco staining on the nails indicative of smoking

Neck

Carotid Pulse

can be observed and palpated - is regular and does not change on respiration. As with other arterial pulses changes indicate cardiac disease *see pulses*.

Jugular Venous Pulse = JVP

This is a venous pulse hence "softer" it can be observed but not palpated. It is irregular with twitching and has a complex wave associated with events in the cardiac cycle.

To measure the JVP place the patient in a supine position at 45° – light from behind and observe the pulsation in the neck – the highest point is the measure of the JVP height above the sternal angle.

1 JVP

2 sternocleidomastoid m

3 Clavicle

When raised >3cm - it indicates RV failure, ± fluid overload.

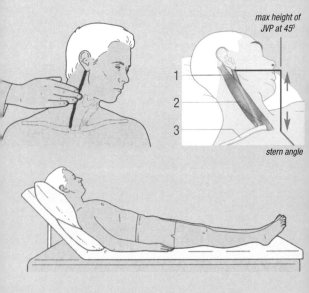

max height of JVP at 45°

stern angle

© A. L. Neill

JVP waveform

a wave = atrial contraction
   absent in atrial fibrillation
   cannon waves = irregular large waves associated with AV
   dissociation
   giant a waves = pulmonary hypertension

c wave = tricuspid valve closure

v wave = end of atrial filling with tricuspid valve closure
   raised in tricuspid valve regurgitation

x wave/ trough = atrial relaxation

y wave / trough = rapid/onset of ventricular filling

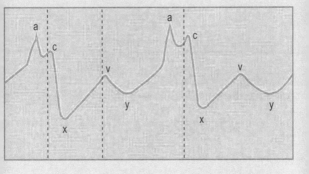

Palpation

Anterior chest wall = Praecordium

Feel the anterior chest wall for the Apex beat - difficult in 20% of patients so tipping the patient over to allows for better sensation –

Apex beat abnormalities

lateral displacement	LV dilatation ± hypertrophy, mediastinal shift
double	LV dyskinesia, V septum hypertrophy, aneurysm
dyskinetic	previous myopathy LV infarction
heaving	LV hypertrophy
tapping = palpable HS1 - mitral stenosis	

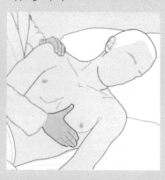

Heart Base abnormalities
Aortic and/or Pulmonary valve abnormalities
Thrills = palpable murmurs, if present these are generally pathological

2 positions to detect parasternal heaves

Parasternal heave   RV hypertrophy *see also Inspection*

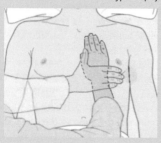

Precussion

The technique of loosely tapping one finger on the body wall to determine the "mass" of the material underneath - although this can be done directly on the patient it is usual to use a base finger and precuss onto this - it is more comfortable for the patient and allows for 2 interpretations of the response - keep nails short to avoid injury and use with auscultation of the area.

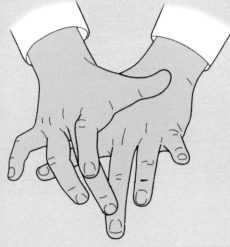

Precussion of the extent of the heart and liver are indicators of CVS disease. Dull areas indicate mass - heart size, fluid accumulation, liver congestion and hollow sounds = hyper-resonant -the extent of the pleural cavity

Pulses

General character of Pulses

Characteristics to look for on the arterial pulse – generally using the radial pulse

Normal rate b/n 60-90/min >90 tachycardia <60 bradycardia regular

normal	Korotoff sound	usual range
collapsing	fast rise and fall	aortic regurgitation Ar atherosclerotic aorta hyperdynamic circulation patent ductus arteriosus
plateau	slow rise	aortic stenosis As
alterans	alternate strong & weak beats	LV failure
pulsus paradoxus	pressure decrease in inspiration >15mmHg	asthma – severe cardiac tamponade
irregular		atrial fibrillation ectopic beats, sinus arrhythmia

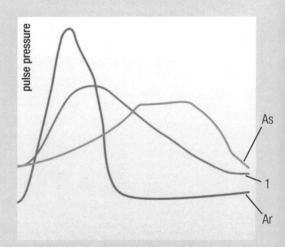

© A. L. Neill

Head & Neck - not usually examined

1 Auricular pulse - in front of the ear near TMJ
2 Carotid pulse - see Inspection
3 Mandibular pulse - under the angle of the jaw
4 Temporal pulse - at the lateral corner of the eye

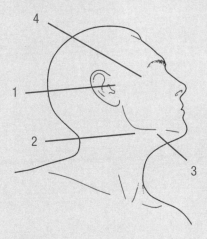

Lower Limb

Dorsalis Pedis – proximal end of the 1st metatarsal space

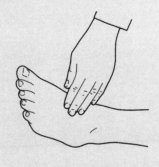

Femoral pulse - just below the inguinal lig and medial to the femoral vein & N. This is the strongest pulse in the body.

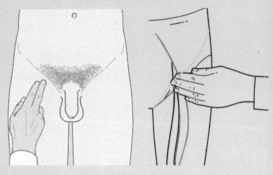

Popliteal pulse - relax the leg and push deep to the hamstrings to compress against the Tibia.

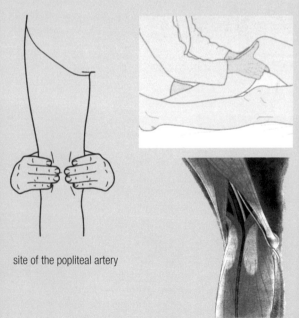

site of the popliteal artery

© A. L. Neill

Posterior Tibial pulse - Site of the posterior tibial artery - in the tarsal tunnel

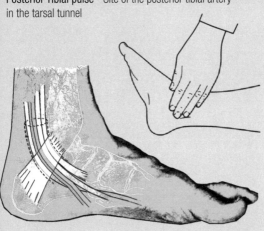

Upper Limb

1 axillary pulse
2 brachial pulse
3 cubital pulse / used for BP measurement
4 radial pulse
5 thumb pulse /anatomical snuff box
6 ulnar pulse

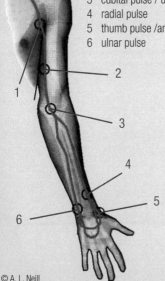

© A. L. Neill

Radial pulse - examining for a collapsing pulse, elevate arm.

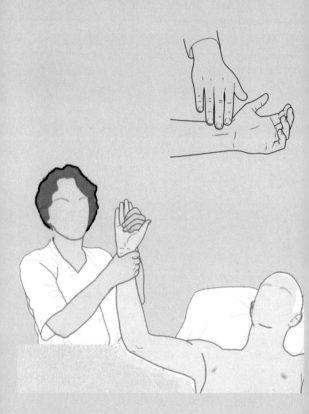

© A. L. Neill

Procedures

Blood Pressure measurement

Measured using a BP cuff of 12.5cm or wider for obese patients in order not to overestimate the levels. The arm should be raised to the level of the heart and the following sounds will be heard. Mercury measures are the most reliable but air pressure valves are commonly used as well as automatic cuffs – which also tend to overestimate the BP levels and need to be calibrated regularly.

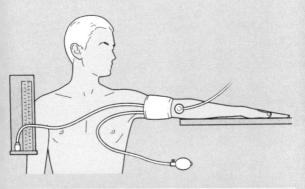

phase		Korotoff sound	usual range
1	KI	thuds / heart beats	120mmHg – systolic P
2	KII	increased volume and blowing noise	110mmHg
3	KIII	softening of thuds	100mmHg
4	KIV	disappearing of regular beats –soft blowing nose	90mmHg
5	KV	no sound	80mmHg – diastolic P

Electrical measurement of cardiac activity

Changes in the activity indicate changes in the conduction through the heart.

The typical ECG reading is associated with particular events of the cardiac cycle.

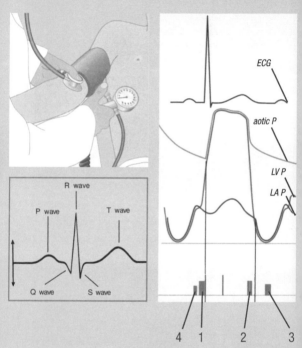

P wave = atrial depolarization

QRS Complex = ventricular depolarization

T wave = ventricular repolarization

HS = 1,2,3,4

© A. L. Neill

Clinical Examination of the Lymph Nodes

Cervical LNs

1 submental
2 submandibular
3 jugular chain
4 supraclavicular – Virchow's
5 post. Triangular
6 postauricular
7 preauricular
8 occipital

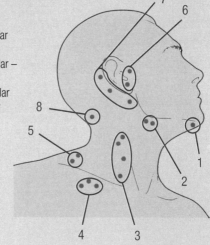

Examination of the epitrochlear node

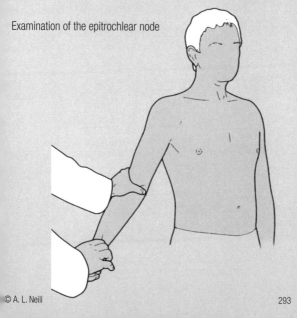

Examination of the Axillary nodes

1 central
2 lateral
3 pectoral
4 infraclavicular
5 subscapular

The 5 groups are best felt with the arm adducted and the fingers pushed deeply into the axilla.

© A. L. Neill

Notes